BIOLOGICAL ACTIVITY
OF NATURAL PRODUCTS

BIOCHEMISTRY RESEARCH TRENDS

BIOLOGICAL ACTIVITY
OF NATURAL PRODUCTS

JAROSLAVA ŠVARC-GAJIĆ

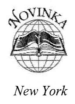

New York

Library of Congress Cataloging-in-Publication Data

ISBN: 978-1-62808-926-4

Published by Nova Science Publishers, Inc. † New York

CONTENTS

Preface   vii

Introduction   ix

Chapter I   **Bioactivity and Toxicity**   **1**
    1. Gastrointestinal Absorption   *6*
    2. Absorption via Respiratory Tract   *6*
    3. Dermal Absorption   *7*
    4. Biotransformation of Xenobiotics   *9*
    5. Toxicodynamics   *11*
    References   *14*

Chapter II   **Natural Bioactive Compounds**   **15**
    1. Traditional Medicine   *15*
    2. Homeopathy   *17*
    3. Chemistry of Natural Compounds   *17*
    4. Isolation of Natural Bioactive Compounds   *25*
    References   *31*

Chapter III   **Medicinal Use of Some Phytochemicals**   **33**
    1. Kava-Kava   *34*
    2. Phenylalanine   *35*
    3. Phytoestrogens   *36*
    4. Psoralens   *37*
    5. Safrole   *38*
    6. Serotonin   *39*
    7. Carotenoids   *41*
    References   *43*

Chapter IV   **Medicinal Use of Alkaloids**   **45**
                    1. Ergot Alkaloids   *45*
                    2. Purine Alkaloids   *49*
                    3. Nux-Vomica Alkaloids   *50*
                    4. Tropane Alkaloids   *52*
                    5. Solanum Alkaloids   *53*
                    References   *55*

Chapter V   **Adverse Effects of Natural Phenols**   **57**
                    1. Major Classes of Natural Phenols   *58*
                    2. Gossypol   *61*
                    3. Phlorizin   *64*
                    4. Resveratrol   *66*
                    5. Hydroxytyrosol   *68*
                    6. Caffeic and Ferulic Acids   *69*
                    7. Antraquinones   *70*
                    References   *71*

Chapter VI   **Risks Associated with Bioactive Food Ingredients**   **75**
                    1. Biogenic Amines   *76*
                    2. Amino-Acid Analogs   *77*
                    3. Bioactive Compounds from Spices   *81*
                    4. Bioactive Compounds from Common Food   *85*
                    References   *91*

Chapter VII   **Medicinal Use of Venoms**   **93**
                    1. Snake Venoms   *94*
                    2. Lizard and Frog Venoms   *98*
                    3. Insect Venoms   *100*
                    4. Venoms of Marine Organisms   *105*
                    5. Antivenoms   *106*
                    References   *109*

Chapter VIII   **Chemometry of Natural Compounds**   **111**
                    1. QSPR Models   *114*
                    2. QSRR Models   *115*
                    3. Lipophilicity in ADME (Absorption, Distribution,
                    Metabolism, Excretion) and QSRR Models   *116*
                    4. In Silico Modeling   *120*
                    References   *131*

Index   **133**

PREFACE

Recognition that various naturally-occurring substances can affect different functions of man and other living organisms came long time ago. In order to exploit biological activity of both natural and synthetic compounds it is important to understand mechanisms underlying effects of different bioactive products.

The book deals with natural bioactive compounds of different origin, including plant, microbial, marine and animal chemicals. Material starts with explanation of bioactivity and basic toxicological principles that are necessary for understanding behavior of xenobiotics upon their entrance in human body. Since natural bioactive compounds were used for millennia by humans, some traditional and alternative medicinal approaches are explained in the book, including Ayurveda, Chinese medicine and homeopathy, as frequently used alternative medical practices today. Because natural sources of bioactive compounds are valuable industrial row materials, technological processes of isolation of several important compounds are elaborated step by step, explaining extraction, isomerization and purification stages at the industrial scale. As examples, technological production processes of ergot and opium alkaloids, as well as bioactive compounds from marine organisms are presented.

Phytochemicals are most readily available and assessable sources of natural bioactive compounds, so material covered by the book deals with some plant chemicals that may exhibit different biological effects, from beneficial to adverse. The use of plants and plant chemicals in traditional medicinal preparations, but also by a modern medicine, are explained.

Alkaloids fall into classes of natural most potent products. The use of ergot, purine, nux-vomica and other alkaloids by modern pharmacology is explained in the book, identifying natural sources and explaining mechanisms of biological effects.

Mostly beneficial health effects have been associated with natural phenols, however under certain circumstances these natural, plant-derived chemicals can exhibit adverse health effects in both humans and animals. After giving classification of natural phenolic compounds, book explains dual character of some natural phenols, focusing on gossypol, phlorizin, resveratrol, hydoxytyrosol, some phenolic acids and antraquinones. In addition, the use of some natural phenols in modern medical practice is explained.

Spices have long been used in different cultures as aphrodisiacs and remedies due to their potent bioactive chemicals. In some specific diets spices can represent an important source of bioactive chemicals and can provoke certain physiological effects. Some fruits, grains, legumes and vegetables also produce physiologically-active compounds and are more probable to provoke biological response due to greater quantities of these dietary products used in comparison to spices.

Today venoms are used as valuable medicinal compounds for both diagnostic and curative purposes. For diagnosis of blood chemistry deficiencies snake venoms are commonly used, whereas improved, non-addictive analgesics are based on cone snail venoms. The book stresses medicinal usability of venoms, produced by different organisms, including insects, marine species, snakes, lizards etc. In addition, biochemistry, production and use of antivenoms are explained.

Chemometry is multidisciplinary scientific discipline heavily used in metabolomics, analytical chemistry, biochemistry, medicine etc. This modern science may be very useful in predicting biological effects of natural products, as well as their derivatives. Since natural products are great inspiration to modern pharmacology, chemometric analysis is indispensable in studying natural bioactive compounds. The book explains basic chemometric principles and most frequently used chemometric models, including QSPR (Quantitative Structure Property Relationship), QSAR (Quantitative Structure Activity Relationship) and QSRR (Quantitative Structure Retention Relationship). Further, the material deals with *in silico* modeling that is used in modern science to define or predict molecular properties or to predict bioactivity, basic pharmacokinetic steps and interaction with receptors.

INTRODUCTION

Natural bioactive products of plant, animal, microbial and mineral origin have been used throughout the history for different purposes, for preparing traditional medicines or as aphrodisiacs and poisons. Bioactive products produced naturally encompass very diverse chemical classes, from simple molecules to highly condensed forms, alkaloids, saponins, peptides, terpenoids etc., playing different roles in producing specie. The effects of some natural products were well recognized and elucidated early in the history, whereas the effects of others remained for a long time mystified and misconcepted. With science development and improvement of analytical tools natural bioactive compounds were able to be accurately identified. Elucidation of natural chemical structures along with advances in organic synthesis made possible the reproduction of natural structures with promising activity. This is particularly important when natural resources are limited or when isolation of certain complex bioactive structures is either economically unviable or extremely complex.

Even though up-to-date thousands of natural bioactive molecules have been discovered, the search for new bioactive molecules from nature continues to occupy numerous scientific disciplines in intention to discover new medicinal agents. Many chemical structures that have been discovered in the nature have an established place in modern pharmacology and today are used as components of approved drugs for different health conditions. In addition to parent chemical structures obtained from nature, numerous pharmaceuticals have been derived from natural molecules by chemical modification. This approach combined with multidisciplinary scientific disciplines, like metabolomics and chemometry, offer extremely wide possibilities in the design of novel pharmaceuticals. Pharmacology for this reason develops rapidly opening a market to new biomolecules. Natural bioactive structures should therefore be considered as never-ending sources of new medicines and valuable drug templates. They are used today to produce pharmaceuticals with improved pharmacokinetic and pharmacodynamic characteristics. In this respect microorganisms, marine organisms, animals and plants, continue to be studied because they all offer wide array of possible structures that can be exploited by humans to produce specific biological effect and targeting particular systems.

Chapter I

BIOACTIVITY AND TOXICITY

Recognition that various naturally-occurring substances can affect different functions of man and other living organisms came long time ago. Several thousand years ago, humans met toxicants of plant, animal and mineral origin. The mechanisms underlying the effects of different bioactive compound are often very complex. Bioactivity is generally dose-dependent, arises via different mechanisms, and it is not uncommon for one compound to exhibit effects ranging from beneficial to adverse.

One of the most important figures in the development of toxicology as scientific discipline was Paracelsus or Auroleus Phillipus Theophrastus Bombastus von Hohenheim. He defined the principles that are still valid and accepted by modern toxicology. Paracelsus considered Galen's principles primitive and lectured in German language, instead in Latin, what was common for the time. He was the first who introduced metals, like mercury and antimony, into medical practice. Antimony pills that he used to treat alcoholism had double effect – mechanical, by provoking peristalsis, and chemical due to emetic properties of antimony oxide that was formed on the surface. Similarly he used to store wine in antimony glasses and to serve it later to alcoholics. In this case antimony-tartrate was responsible for nausea in consumers and emetic effect. By using *Quinta essentia vini*, or wine essence, obtained by wine distillation, Paracelsus produced the essence of animal, plant and mineral row materials. The procedure represented, in fact, extraction with ethanol obtained by wine distillation. *Quinta essentia* of bismuth, different salts, pearls, flowers, camphor, seeds, horns and other materials were used by him for treating different health conditions. The strongest contribution of Paracelsus to modern toxicology, however, was the awareness of the dose significance. He claimed that every substance is toxic and that only dose determines whether the toxic effect will be expressed or not.

Bioactive substance can provoke systematic effects only after it has been absorbed and transferred into the blood. Local effects occur as a result of direct interactions on a contact site, such as on the skin in dermal contact, or in the respiratory organs immediately upon inhalation. Some substances may express both local and systematic toxic effects. For example, tetraethyl lead is readily absorbed via dermal route, leaving the skin wounds and provoking systematic effects soon after absorption, particularly profound in CNS. After absorption, the effects can be expressed on specific organs and systems, such as gastrointestinal, respiratory or cardiovascular, or may affect entire organism by affecting e.g. a nervous system.

Toxicant molecules and particles while finding their way to the blood are confronted to many barriers such as skin or mucosal membranes. Each tissue level barrier is composed of numerous subbarriers on a cellular level and chemical has to pass cell membranes for many times in order to reach systematic circulation. The resistance to molecule entrance into the cell varies for neutral molecules of a different size and for charged ions. As a part of body's protective mechanism, the transport of toxicants into certain sensitive tissues, such as brain or developing fetus, can be hindered by specific body barriers, such as placental or blood/brain barrier. Blood/brain barrier is not completely developed in newborns, making them more susceptible to toxicant influence. This is a reason for morphine being 10 times more toxic to newborn rats in comparison to adults (Švarc-Gajić, 2009).

Upon entering the blood the substances bind to plasma proteins. Highly lipophylic substances are further transported via lymph. Albumin (Figure I.1) is one of the most abundant plasma proteins and it readily binds Ca, Cu, Zn, bilirubin, vitamin C, antibiotics, histamine, barbiturates and other substances. Transfferin, which is actually a β1-globulin, binds iron and transports it throughout the body. Ceruroplasmine (α2-globulin) is responsible for copper binding, while α- and β-lipoproteins bind lipophylic substances, steroid hormones, cholesterol, vitamins, etc. (Švarc-Gajić, 2009).

In first stages of toxicant distribution, most affected organs are organs which are the most vascularized, such as liver, kidneys, lungs and glands. Poorly vascularized tissues, such as fat tissue or muscles, takeover only small part of the toxicant. In later stages of the distribution the role of circulation decreases and the retention of the compound by the tissue depends mostly on the chemical affinity. Immediately upon absorption lead, for example, is highest in erythrocytes, kidneys and liver. After a month, most of the remaining lead is stored in bone tissue. Liver and kidneys have high capacity for various chemicals due to high concentration of intracellular proteins.

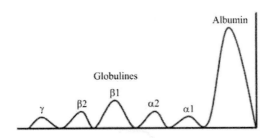

Figure I.1. Plasma proteins separated by electrophoresis.

The existence of blood/brain barrier that limits the entrance of substances from blood into the brain was first observed in experiments in the late 19th century when it was noticed that if aniline dye is injected into the blood all tissues except the brain become stained. Later on the reverse experiment in which the dye was injected into the spinal fluid, staining only the brain, confirmed the existence of such barrier. Blood vessels in the brain are not in direct contact with the tissue, but are covered with the layer of specific endothelial cells. Endothelial cells comprise only 0.1% of the brain weight, but they make about 644 km long line, with a surface area of 20 m^2 (Švarc-Gajić, 2009).Tight junctions between endothelial cells (Figure I.2) prevent free entrance of foreign substances. In addition, endothelial cells metabolize certain molecules to prevent their entry into the central nervous system. For example, L-DOPA, the precursor to dopamine, can cross the blood-brain barrier, and is further metabolized to dopamine. Precursor thus, is used to treat dopamine-deficient patients. Glial cells surrounding capillaries in the brain, as well as low concentration of interstitial proteins in the brain, prevent access of hydrophilic molecules. However some smaller molecules, like alcohol, caffeine and nicotine, are easily transferred into the brain.

Distribution of xenobiotics from systematic circulation to fetal tissue is also limited. Placenta has a very large surface area, which facilitates the transport of essential substances, as well as metabolic products in both directions. The surface area at term is approximately 11 m^2 and about 5 to 10% of placental surface is only few micrometers thin (Švarc-Gajić, 2009).

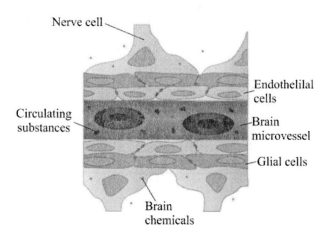

Figure I.2. Blood-brain barrier.

Intervillous filled with mothers blood

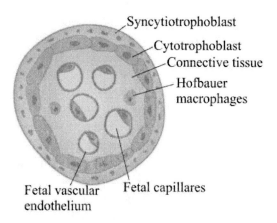

Figure I.3. Placental barrier.The structure of villus, functional unit of human placenta.

Exchange between maternal and fetal circulating substances takes place in chorionic villus, which is the functional unit of human placenta (Figure I.3). There are about 150 ml of maternal blood in the intervillous space. Villi are covered with trophoblastic cells, important in the formation of placental barrier. Trophoblastic cells are present as mononuclear cells called cytotrophoblasts and multinucleate cells, syncytiotrophoblast. In addition to trophoblast layer fetal and maternal circulations are separated by the connective tissue space, endothelial basement membrane and fetal capillary endothelium.

Substances can be absorbed via different routes, however most frequent are oral, dermal and respiratory. Resorptive surface area of the gastrointestinal tract is around 300 m^2 and most significant absorption occurs in small intestine even though some compounds are well absorbed from the stomach. A finger-like structures of gut mucose vili (Figure I.4), give surface area to small intestine of a 500-600 m long tube (Švarc-Gajić, 2009).

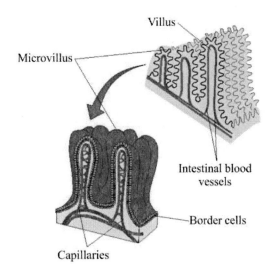

Figure I.4. Inner surface of small intestine.

In other routes of exposure, such as dermal or intravenous, the substance avoids so called first-pass effect or intense metabolism in the liver, and is usually more toxic. Consequently, the toxicity and behavior of xenobiotics are highly dependent on the route of entry. Snake venoms are for these reasons toxic only after intravenous injection, whereas in gastrointestinal tract they become inactivated by metabolic transformation, mostly taking place in the liver.

1. GASTROINTESTINAL ABSORPTION

Majority of toxicants are resorbed from gut by simple diffusion and in this process the degree of lipophylic character determines the rate of absorption. A dose of hydrophilic character is required for good absorption in order to provide a good contact with resorptive surface, i.e. a hydrophilic mucose. Absorption in gastrointestinal tract is favorable when acidity converts the molecule to unionized form. Consequently, acidic conditions in small intestine favor the absorption of acidic substances, while alkaline conditions, like those in large intestine, support the absorption of the alkaline substances.

Many factors influence gut absorption, such as peristaltic activity, particle size, aggregate state, etc. Proteins and other food components may sorb the toxicant in the gastrointestinal tract reducing its bioavailability. Bacterial enzymes which catalyze hydrolytic and reductive reactions take a part in biotransformation of xenobiotics and can activate or inactivate many toxic substances. Children are more susceptible to methemoglobinemia due to undeveloped *Escherichia coli* which, in this case, doesn't perform reductive reactions efficiently and allows more food nitrates to oxidize hemoglobin. Beneficial activity of gut flora includes reduction of aromatic nitro and amino organic compounds, which often express carcinogenic or goitrogenic activity. Cyanide glycosides, present in kernel of many fruits, like peach and apricot, can be hydrolyzed to very toxic cyanides by microbial enzymes, increasing their toxicity.

2. ABSORPTION VIA RESPIRATORY TRACT

Toxicants in the form of gases, vapors or solid particles may enter respiratory system and can be absorbed in different ways, depending on their physico-chemical properties. Gases and vapors follow the same route in the lungs as inhaled air during normal breathing. The route of solid particles is somewhat different and depends significantly on a particle size.

Absorption via respiratory tract may be very efficient due to large resorptive surface of 50-100 m^2 and 600 millions of alveoli in lungs where transfer to the blood takes place. In addition, the walls of alveoli and capillaries are extremely thin (1-2 μm) making the transfer of substances rapid. Alveoli are surrounded by a network of thin-walled capillaries (Figure I.5) and only about 0.2 µm separates alveoli from capillaries (Švarc-Gajić, 2009).Mucus that moistures alveoli walls enhance lung absorption.

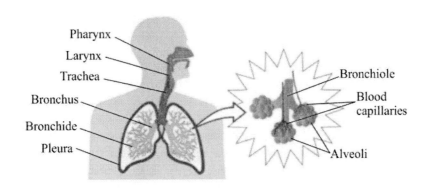

Figure I.5. Respiratory tract.

Fate of solid particles that entered the lungs depends on a particle diameter. Particles smaller than 0.1 µm are expelled with the turbulent current of exhaled air, whereas particles in the diameter range 0.1-1 µm reach alveoli (Švarc-Gajić, 2009). Larger particles are retained on the epithelium of the nose and trachea. Soluble particles can be absorbed from these compartments of respiratory tract after their dissolution. Insoluble particles are mostly expelled by the movement of ciliated epithelium. Expelled toxicant particles can enter mouth and can be swallowed, following the route of gastrointestinal absorption. Phagocyted particles are partially removed by excreted mucilage, however some amount can enter lymph nodes. The deposition of solid particles in lungs can permanently damage lung tissue and may provoke pneumoconiosis. Inorganic materials, such as coal, silica, HgO, asbestos, and plant dust, are particularly dangerous in this respect.

3. DERMAL ABSORPTION

Consideration of dermal absorption is important in many occupational exposures. Skin makes 15% of the human body weight and is the largest organ of the human body with surface area of 1.5-2.0 m^2 (Švarc-Gajić, 2009). Skin has a complex role in human body protecting it from mechanical injury, providing the sensation and regulating the temperature. Skin`s immune system is a natural defense barrier against microorganisms and is associated with SALT (skin associated lymphoid tissue). Lymphoid epidermal cells are also involved in delayed hypersensitivity reactions, or contact dermatitis. Synthesis of vitamins D and B that occurs in the skin is linked to pigmentation. Skin may be important portal of entry of foreign compounds, as well as mean of their excretion.

The structure of the skin is quite complex (Figure I.6). Older dermal cells are pushed to the surface by new cells which are produced in germinative layer at the border of epidermis and dermis, becoming filled with keratin. This keratinized layer (*stratum corneum*) can absorb water representing an important part of hydrophilic-lipophylic barrier that skin presents. Rather complex composition of the cornified cells in *stratum corneum* provides a strong chemical resistance. Lipophylic part of skin's barrier arises from excreted lipids and waxes from various glands, embedded in the dermis.

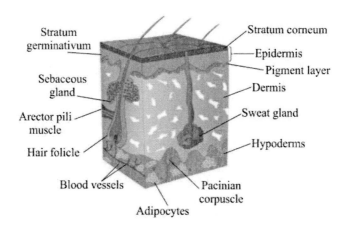

Figure I.6. The structure of the skin.

Water absorbed by keratinized layer can significantly enhance the entrance of toxic substances through opened pores and gland tubules. Lipophylic toxicants are absorbed by diffusion through many cell layers. Dermally well absorbed are low molecular weight, non-charged, hydrophobic substances.

Depending on the skin thickness, absorption of a given substance at different body skin parts varies. For example, hydrocortisone is absorbed over

50 times more by genital skin in comparison to the skin of the palms (Švarc-Gajić, 2009). With aging skin becomes thinner, less elastic and more easily damaged, receiving less blood flow and expressing lower gland activity. Chemical substance can be activated or transformed in the skin by the energy of ultraviolet radiation and can provoke photosensitive or photoallergic reactions.

4. BIOTRANSFORMATION OF XENOBIOTICS

The toxicity of certain xenobiotic is highly influenced by the body's ability to metabolize and excrete the compound. Enzymes, involved in biotransformation processes of foreign compounds were developed as a result of evolutionary adaptation. Biotransformation occurs in two phases. In phase I reactions a polar group is introduced into the molecule, or the polar group is unmasked. These reactions usually prepare the compound for the reactions of conjugation with some endogenous molecules that occurs in the second phase. Phase II reactions are, thus, the reactions of synthesis requiring energy and this is provided by ATP. Most of enzymes involved in phase I reactions are bound to the membrane of endoplasmatic reticulum. Enzymes, catalyzing phase II reactions, are mostly located in the cytosolic fraction.

Important family of phase I oxidation enzymes are *cytochrome P450 oxidases*. The enzymes contain a hem group at the active site. When hem iron is reduced with sodium dithionyl and complexed with carbon monoxide, formed colored product shows the absorbance at 450 nm, thus the enzymes were named accordingly. Cytochrome P450 oxidases metabolize multiple substrates, and many enzymes in the family can catalyze multiple reactions. Their role is important in hormone synthesis and breakdown, cholesterol synthesis and vitamin D metabolism.

Flavin-containing monooxygenase system (FMO) group of oxidation enzymes contain flavin adenine dinucleotide as a cofactor (Figure I.7). These enzymes make microsomal fraction of cellular proteins and many isoenzymes of this family are known. Major difference between this system and the cytochrome P450 monooxygenase system, is that the FMO system does not oxidize carbon atoms, however many reactions catalyzed by FMO can also be catalyzed by cytochrome P450. In contrast to P450 monooxygenase system, the FMO system cannot be induced.

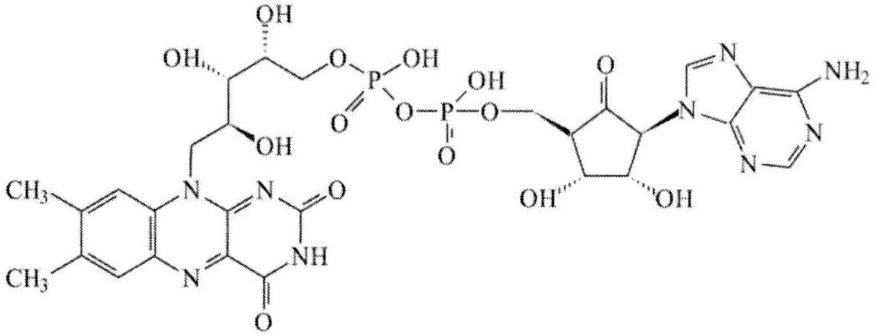

Figure I.7. Flavin adenine dinucleotide (FAD), a cofactor of FMO enzyme system.

Evolutionary purpose of *alcohol dehydrogenases* was probably the inactivation of alcohols naturally occurring in foods or produced by bacteria in the gastrointestinal tract. Metabolism of primary alcohols, catalyzed by enzymes, is faster in comparison to secondary and tertiary alcohols. In yeast and many bacteria, this class of enzymes catalyzes the opposite reaction, i.e. alcohol synthesis in fermentation process. Six different alcohol dehydrogenases were identified in humans (Švarc-Gajić, 2009). All of them are dimmers having a zinc ion in their active centre which plays an important role for fixing the hydroxyl group of alcohols in place at the catalytic site. Short-chain alcohol dehydrogenases containing calcium or magnesium are involved mostly in the metabolism of secondary alcohols. In yeasts alcohol dehydrogenases are tetramers.

Monoamine oxygenases (MAO) contain covalently-bound cofactor flavin-adenine-dinucleotide (FAD). The enzymes are bound to the outer membrane of mitochondria and are involved in the destruction of biogenic amines, such as serotonin, adrenaline, noradrenalin and others. There are two types of MAO enzymes, of type A and B and both are found in neurons. MAO dysfunction is linked to depression, aggression, attention deficit disorder and social phobias (Švarc-Gajić, 2009).

Reductive reactions are performed in anaerobic conditions with the implication of nicotine amide adenine dinucleotide (NADH) or NADPH cofactors. Mammals have a poor ability to reduce compounds because their tissues and body fluids are oxygenated, however intestinal bacteria may contribute to reduction reaction and to inactivation of many xenobiotics. *Peroxidases*, hem containing enzymes, catalyze the destruction of dangerous organic peroxides. The enzymes are active with both hydrogen peroxides and organic hydroperoxides, such as lipid peroxides. Glutathione peroxidase is a peroxidase found in humans, which contains selenocysteine. It uses glutathione, an endogenous tripeptide, as an electron donor. *Hydrolytical enzymes* are located mostly in plasma and various tissues, where they constitute both microsomal and cytosolic fractions. Hydroxylation of aren oxides as well as aliphatic and aromatic peroxides, dangerous due to their high reactivity with body nucleophiles (DNA, proteins), is catalyzed by these reactions.

Phase II reactions are usually catalyzed by enzymes involving various cofactors which react with polar functional groups belonging to parent compounds or introduced into molecules by phase I reactions. Glucuronides are the most common conjugates of toxicants that are excreted in bile. Glucuronide conjugates are often subjected to hydrolysis by gut β-glucuronidases (hydrolases), prolonging the residence time of the toxicant. In toxicology this is known as enterohepatic circulation. Sulfate esters, produced by sulfatation reactions, are completely ionized and are, thus, easily excreted in urine. Methyl conjugates are generally less hydrophilic than parent compounds, nevertheless these reaction are considered to be detoxification reaction. In acylation reactions carboxylic group of xenobiotic is conjugated with amino group of endogenous aminoacids, such as glycine, glutamine, arginine, taurine or ornithine (birds, reptiles). In order to be conjugated, the compound requires previous activation with acetyl-CoA.

5. TOXICODYNAMICS

5.1. Interaction with Receptors

Receptors receive chemical, electromagnetic, as well as mechanical stimuli, producing a chemical signal that is further transmitted through the cell. These important cell proteins can be studied by X-ray crystallography, NMR or by computer modeling. Ligands that can activate receptors are peptides, small molecules (neurotransmitters, hormones), xenobiotics (drugs), toxins and others. Upon ligand binding to the receptors membrane potential changes, initiating a signal. In many hormonal disorders, elevated or insufficient production of certain hormone isn't always a real cause of the illness. In the core of the disorder may be a genetic defect with hereditable impaired receptor genes. Hormonal levels in the body can be normal and endocrine disorder can arise as a result of nonfunctional receptors. Body self-regulates receptor functions by changing the number of available receptors. At high insulin plasma concentrations, for example, the number of surface receptors for insulin is gradually reduced by endocytosis of insulin-receptor complexes and subsequent intracellular liposomal activity. The synthesis of new hormone receptors occurs in endoplasmatic reticulum.

Receptors are, in fact, peripheral or integral membrane proteins. Many transmembrane receptors are composed of two or more protein subunits which dissociate upon ligand binding. Transmembrane domain of the receptor is mostly composed of alpha helix, and may contain a ligand binding pocket. Transmembrane receptors can further be divided to ionotropic and metabotropic. Ionotropic receptors are ligand-gated ion channels that open and close in response to ligand, allowing a flow of ions that changes the membrane potential. Metabotropic receptors are coupled to G-proteins and affect cell indirectly through enzymes which control the opening of ion channels. Intracellular receptors are found on membranes of organelles, a nucleus or are free in the cytoplasm. Receptors of steroidal hormones like estrogen, androgen, progesterone, glucocorticosteroids, mineralocorticosteroids, as well as for thyroid hormones, fall into this group. Complex formed between the ligand and the intracellular receptor may enter the cell nucleus modulating gene expression. Retinoid receptors are intracellular receptors and vitamin A is a known teratogen, indicating that in the core of teratogenesis may be a modulated gene expression.

Ligands that activate their innate receptors are known as *agonists*, whereas *antagonists* disrupt ligand interaction with receptors inhibiting the function of agonists. In poisoning treatment antagonists have important role as antidotes blocking the effects of toxins. *Competitive antagonists* don't induce any biological response by themselves, whereas *inverse antagonists* bind to the active site, but produce distinct set of biological responses. *Non-competitive antagonists* bind to a distinctly separate binding site, different of that of the agonist, perturbing the activity of receptors. Once bound to receptors, non-competitive antagonists may decrease the affinity for agonist on particular receptor, or may prevent conformational changes required for receptor activation. Many antagonists are *reversible antagonists* that, like most agonists, bind and unbind to receptors at rates determined by receptor-ligand kinetics. *Irreversible antagonists* covalently bind to receptor target and, generally, cannot be removed. The receptor in such situations is inactivated until new receptors are synthetized. *Partial agonists* compete with full agonists for active site on the receptor and act as competitive antagonists if they are co-administrated.

5.2. Toxicokinetics

The kinetics of toxicant elimination can be defined by monitoring the decay in plasma levels of the toxicant. In theoretical one-compartment open model the distribution of the compound from plasma to other tissues and organs is neglected. For such approximation an exponential decay of toxicant plasma concentration may be observed due to saturation of the excretory system. Such dependence indicates that different amounts of the substance are excreted in equal time intervals. Knowledge on the functional dependence allows the calculation of the toxicant concentration in tissues, assuming that plasma and tissue concentrations are equal. Most toxicants are eliminated via first order kinetics.

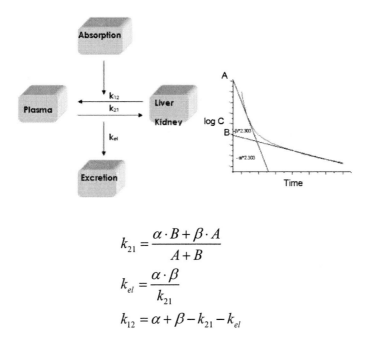

$$k_{21} = \frac{\alpha \cdot B + \beta \cdot A}{A + B}$$

$$k_{el} = \frac{\alpha \cdot \beta}{k_{21}}$$

$$k_{12} = \alpha + \beta - k_{21} - k_{el}$$

Figure I.8. Two-compartment open model.

In two-compartment open model toxicant entrance, distribution between plasma and tissues, and excretion take place. Elimination kinetics in such system may be described as an exponential curve on a semilogarithmic scale. Elimination rate changes in the course of time and in this process a rapid (A) and a slow (B) phase are observed (Figure I.8). The values of k_{12}, k_{21} k_{el} constants express the relative influence of the distribution and elimination on a concentration profile.

REFERENCES

Švarc-Gajić J. *General Toxicology*. Nova Science Publishers, New York, 2009.

Chapter II

NATURAL BIOACTIVE COMPOUNDS

Natural bioactive compounds typically occur in small quantities in food, plants, animals and microorganisms. The number of bioactive compounds that have been discovered and identified is quite vast. These compounds are being intensively studied by different scientific disciplines to evaluate their effects on human health. Chemically, natural bioactive compounds are very diverse. Polyketides and fatty acids are composed of acetate units, whereas natural terpenoids and steroids are composed of isoprene units oriented in head and tail manner. Further on, bioactive phenylpropanoids, alkaloids, aminoacids or specialized carbohydrates, are common in nature.

1. TRADITIONAL MEDICINE

Traditional or folk medicine is being practiced for thousands of years and refers to ways of restoring health by means different of those used by modern medicine. Folk medicine is generally transmitted orally through a community or family and in many parts of the World it enjoys great popularity and acceptance. In some Asian and African countries up to 80% of population depends on traditional medicine for primary health care and more than 100 countries have regulations for herbal medicines. In China, traditional herbal medicine accounts for 30% to 50% of total medicinal consumption.

Ayurvedic medicine is a system of traditional medicine native to India that relies on the principle of five elements: air, water, sky, fire and the human body; the principle of seven primary constituent elements: flesh, fat, marrow, bone, blood plasma, semen and female reproductive organs; as well as the principle of elemental energies: air and space; fire and water; water and earth. It is considered that each human possesses a unique combination of energies that defines the person's character and features. Ayurvedic practitioners approach diagnosis by using all five senses. In India, over 100 colleges offer degrees in traditional Ayurvedic medicine.

Siddha medicine is a folk medicine about 10 000 years old that relies on principles close to Ayurveda. This medical system is considered to be perfect because it is believed that it was transmitted to humans by the Hindu God Shiva and the Goddess Parvathi. Remedies used in Siddha are produced from natural products of different origin and have a very complex composition so some may include more than 250 components.

Unani medicine is practiced in South Asia and refers to tradition of Greco-Arabic medicine that arrived in India in 12th-13th century. First compiled writing referring to Unani appeared in 1025 AD. This medical system is based on the teachings of Greek physician Hippocrates, and Roman physician Galen, and was developed to elaborate medical systems of Arabs, Afghans and Persians. Similarly as Ayurveda this medical system is based on four elements related to human body – fire, water, earth and air, and the treatment is highly dependent on diagnosis. In India there are about 40 Unani medical colleges.

Traditional Chinese medicine started with Shang dynasty in the 14th -11th centuries BC. Besides rich herbal medicine, where more than 10 000 medicinal recipes are known, traditional Chinese medicine deals with acupuncture, massage and dietary therapy. Phytotherapy represents a dominant field in the Chinese medicine, however traditional Chinese medical preparations integrate also animal parts, like tiger penis, rhinoceros horns, gallstones, turtles, seahorses, snake oil, bear bile; as well as human parts, like nails, hair, dandruff, earwax, sweat, urine, feces, organs and bones.

In *Mongolian medicine* every plant is believed to be medicinal, as well as pure water. Moxibustion was developed in Mongolia and later on it was incorporated into Tibetan medicine. The procedure represents burning of the mugwort over acupuncture points. The traditional Tibetan medical system is in fact the synthesis of the Ayurveda, Unani, indigenous Tibetan, and Chinese medical systems, and is practiced in Tibet, India, Nepal, Bhutan, Siberia, China and Mongolia, and more recently in some parts of Europe and North America.

2. HOMEOPATHY

The idea of homeopathy was exploited already in 400 B.C. by Hippocrates who prescribed mandrake root to treat mania. Paracelsus in 16th century postulated that "what makes a man ill also cures him" which is the idea of modern homeopathy. Practitioners of homeopathy treat patients using highly diluted solutions of active compounds that are believed to cause healthy people to exhibit symptoms that are similar to those seen in patients. The basic idea of homeopathy, or low of similars: *similia similibus curentur*, was postulated in 1796 by Samuel Hahnemann who used drugs to induce symptoms similar to those of illness. He believed that artificial symptoms would stimulate the vital force of the body helping the recovery process.

Today more than 3000 remedies of animal, plant, mineral origin, as well as numerous synthetic substances are used as homeopathic remedies. Some of common homeopathic ingredients include arsenic oxide, table salt, venoms, thyroid hormone, opium; whereas less common and more specific ingredients may include materials from diseased or pathological products such as fecal, urinary, and respiratory discharges, blood, and tissues. Homeopathic remedies are produced by highly diluting the substance with alcohol or distilled water. In dilutions logarithmic scales are used: X scale for dilution factor of 10, C scale for dilution factor of 100, etc. (Ernst, 2002). Principal question of dispute and controversy in homeopathy is linked to the dose/response relationship. Since homeopaths use dilutions that are not producing sufficient concentrations to cause any effect, in fact, dilutions are often made until no molecule is left, the question on the efficiency of such preparations remains the subject of debates. Such approach is completely in collision with basic pharmacokinetic/toxicokinetic principles.

3. CHEMISTRY OF NATURAL COMPOUNDS

3.1. Bioactive Compounds of Plant Origin

Natural bioactive compounds have been used for millennia in medical practice, but today they are superseded by pharmacological approach. Natural compounds are, however, often the prototypes of biologically active molecules with enhanced pharmacological characteristics and sources of novel medicinal compounds. To support this fact it is important to mention that 40% of medicines have their origin in natural products. The chemistry of natural bioactive compounds, their synthesis and biosynthesis are, therefore, major areas of organic chemistry today. By derivatizing natural bioactive molecules pharmacological properties, such as efficiency, water solubility, chemical stability, and toxicity, can by optimized.

A number of plant *steroids* demonstrate useful pharmacological activity. These include digitalis glycosides (cardenolides) which are used in the treatment of heart failure, steroidal alkaloids that occur in plants of *Solanaceae* family, steroidal saponins and others. About 30 cardiotonic glycosides were isolated from *Digitalis purpurea*. Mexican yam is a plant rich in steroidal saponin diosgenin that is used as a starting material for synthesis of steroidal hormones.

Cyanogenic glycosides are produced by plants of Fabaceae, Rosaceae, Linaceae and Compositae families, and are concentrated in kernels and seeds of many fruits like cherries, plums, almonds, peaches, apricots and apples. The amount of the produced glycoside depends on the plants age, the variety of the plant, and environmental factors. When ingested they undergo hydrolysis, catalyzed by gut bacteria, releasing hydrogen cyanide, one of the most potent neurotoxins. Cassava is a woody shrub native to South America that is important source of carbohydrates for humans and animals, however it contains significant amounts of cyanogenic glycosides. The content of these glycosides may reach 1 g/kg in the plants root. 100 g of cassava root produces approximately 53 mg of hydrogen cyanide (Švarc-Gajić, 2011). Cassava is detoxified by soaking, cooking or fermentation. Cyanide, released in gastrointestinal tract, rapidly inhibits oxidative processes in cells provoking their death. Average enzymatic capacity in humans that can metabolize toxic glycosides, is about 10 mg of cyanides per hour. Chronic ingestion of cyanogenic glycosides leads to neuropathy, pathological changes in peripheral nervous system, and liver damage, whereas acute poisoning is accompanied with chest and throat tightness, nausea, muscle weakness, and mental confusion (Švarc-Gajić, 2011).

Coumarin is abundant in cassia (*Cinnamomum aromaticum*) bark which is one of the four components of the cinnamon spice. In plants coumarin plays insecticidal role protecting the plants from harmful insects. The compound has a very pleasant and distinctive odor and sweet scent for what it is extensively used in food and pharmaceutical industry. Naturally occurring coumarin is dangerous only when ingested in high amounts or if consumed during prolonged period of time. Warfarin, a synthetic substance related to natural coumarin, is a common anticoagulant and is widely used both as a rodenticide and as a therapeutic agent. Coumarin is not very toxic *per se*, however in moldy hay more dangerous dimmer dicoumarol is formed (Figure II.1) (Švarc-Gajić, 2011). Some beneficial effects of coumarin, such as fungicidal properties and anti-tumor activity, as well as appetite suppressing properties, are currently being investigated.

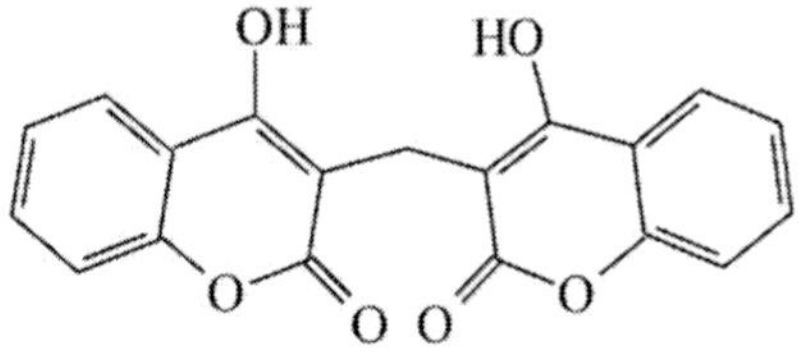

Figure II.1. Dicoumarol.

Estragole is present in essential oils of many spices and has been also identified in pine oil and turpentine, where it contributes to build-up of characteristic strong and sweet flavor. Herbal oils containing estragole have been long used in folk medicine. Today estragole is used for aromatherapy, in perfume industry and as a food additive. Recent concerns about potential carcinogenicity of estragole have led a number of regulatory bodies to call for restrictions on the use of herbs that contain this constituent. Carcinogenicity of the compound has been confirmed in *in vitro* assays and was shown to occur via mutagenic mechanism. Estragole is metabolized to 1'- hydroxyestragole and several epoxides which are further sulfated in hepatocytes. Formed sulfate conjugates readily bind to DNA provoking carcinogenesis in hepatocytes (Švarc-Gajić, 2011). Skin whitening effects of estragole opened a new perspectives concerning estragole role in dermatology.

Pokeweeds belong to *Phytolacca* genus and are indigenous to North America, South America, East Asia and New Zealand. The plant grows up to 3 m and produces dark berries. Active compounds are present in all parts of the plant, but are mostly concentrated in the root. The plant produces several active compounds: an alkaloid phytolaccine; a resin phytolaccotoxin, and a saponin phytolaccigenin (Švarc-Gajić, 2011). Pokeweeds are used in America for salad preparation. Berries and leaves are boiled becoming edible. The leaves of the pokeweeds are prepared as spinach. Double boiling of the leaves and cooking of the berries ensures the breakdown of toxins.

In folk medicine different parts of the pokeweeds are used as emetic, cathartic or narcotic. The root, as a part with the highest content of active compounds, is used to treat conjunctivitis, chronic rheumatism, skin diseases and bowel paralysis. Ingestion of uncooked parts of pokeweed provokes nausea, vomiting, episodes of muscle weakness and spasms, and severe convulsions. In severe poisoning cases death occurs due to respiratory arrest (Švarc-Gajić, 2011).

In *marihuana* (*Cannabis sativa*) more than 60 cannabinoids have been identified with D9-THC-(-)-D9-trans-tetrahydrocannabinol being a major euphoriant. Chemically, cannabinoids represent hybrids between a terpenoid and a phenol, for what they and are sometimes called terpenophenolics. Synthetic D9-THC (dronabinol) was approved by the FDA for the treatment of anorexia associated with weight loss in AIDS patients. Disadvantages of pharmacological use of dronabinol are poor water solubility, undesirable effects on central nervous system, and potential for tolerance, for what another synthetic derivative, nabilone (Figure II.2), was created. In medical practice Nabilone is used for the treatment of nausea and vomiting associated with chemotherapy.

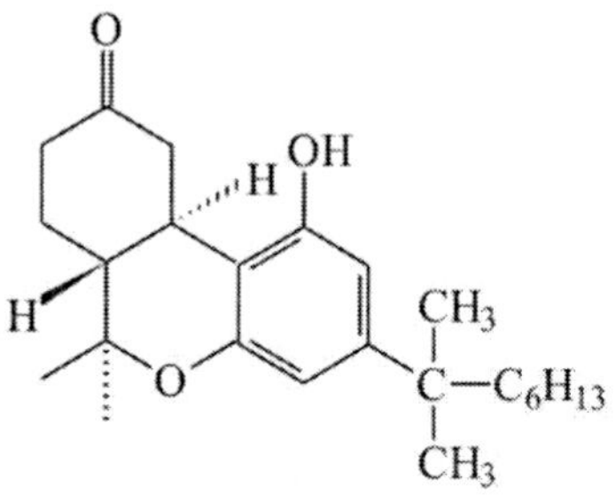

Figure II.2. Nabilone.

Ginkgo (*Ginkgo biloba* L.) is a very old tree indigenous to Chine that is believed to have survived the glace age. The fossils of ginkgo 270 million years old have been discovered and several ginkgo trees survived Hiroshima nuclear blast in 1945. The tree produces nut-like seeds that are highly appreciated in Asiatic cuisine and are believed to have aphrodisiac properties.

Ginkgolides A, B, C, and M (Figure II.3) produced by tree leaves inhibit platelet-aggregating factor (PAF) (Leistner and Drewke, 2010). PAF in addition to its effects on blood platelets causes bronchoconstriction, cutaneous vasodilatation, hypotension, and releases inflammatory mediators in the body.

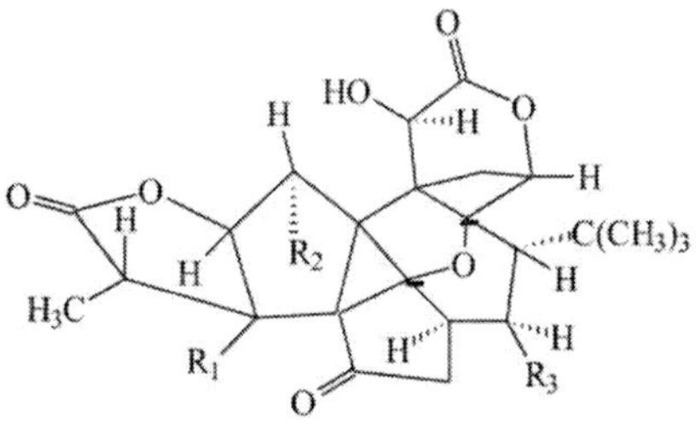

Ginkgolide	R1	R2	R3
A	OH	H	H
B	OH	OH	H
C	OH	OH	OH
J	OH	H	OH
M	H	OH	OH

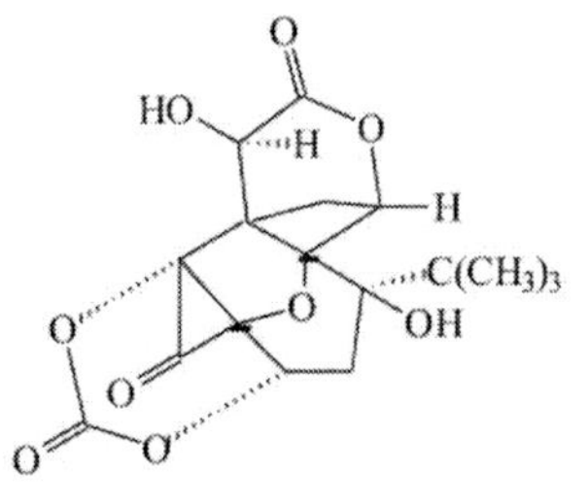

Figure II.3. Ginkgolides from *Ginkgo biloba*.

Certain flavonoid glycosides isolated from ginkgo reduce capillary fragility acting beneficially in the prevention of ischemic brain damage. Gingko components exhibit antioxidant effects via free-radical scavenging, the property important in the protection of blood vessel wall integrity. Analog of vitamin B6, ginkgotoxin (Figure II.4), was first found in trace quantities in leaves of the plant, but later on it was established that the compound is more prevalent in seeds. Ginkgotoxin has an antivitamin effect in mammals, causing symptoms of vitamin B6 deficiency, including loss of consciousness, tonic/clonic seizures, and/or death in very severe cases (Leistner and Drewke, 2010). It is estimated that one would have to consume at least 50 g of ginkgo seeds for such effects to occur.

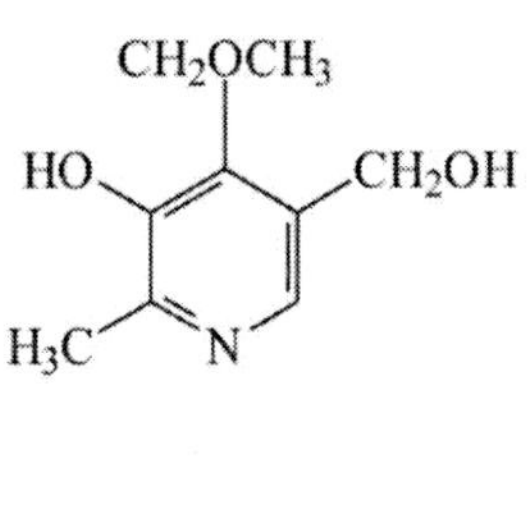

Figure II.4. Ginkgotoxin.

3.2. Bioactive Compounds of Microbial Origin

Microorganisms are sources of numerous bioactive compounds, among which the most well-known and best studied are antibiotics and alkaloids. Probiotics refer to living microorganisms that, following ingestion, form a part of colonic flora, temporarily, improving the health of the host. Various strains, such as *Lactobacillus* and bifidobacteria, are often used in combination as probiotics in the treatment of intestinal infections and diarrhea.

An anaerobic bacterium, *Clostridium botulinum*, has an established place in clinical practice, due to its ability to cause temporary muscle paralysis. Bacterial toxin, a Botulinum toxin, is used in the treatment of dystonic torticollis, blepharospasm, muscle spasms following stroke, anal fissures and achalasia. Dystonic torticollis is characterized by neck muscles contracting involuntarily, causing abnormal movements and awkward posture, whereas blepharospasm refers to involuntary contractions of the muscles around the eyes. Achalasia is characterized with the difficulties to swallow due to incomplete esophagus contraction and relaxation.

Several microbial bioactive compounds have been identified as blood triglyceride lowering agents beneficial in the prevention of cardiovascular diseases. Lovastatin is produced by a fungus (*Aspergillus tereus*) which is used at the industrial scale to produce organic acids. The compounds is also abundantly founds in edible oyster mushrooms (2.8%) and red yeast rice, a rice fermented with the mold *Monascus purpureus*. Similar compound, Pravastatin, has been isolated from Nocardia bacterium. A synthetic derivative Simvastin, was produced based on the identified structures of lovastatin and pravastatin, and nowadays it has an established place in medicine as a blood triglyceride-lowering agent.

A macrolide lactone with immunomodulating properties was isolated from *Streptomyces tsukubaensis*. Isolated compound served as a drug model for Tacrolimus (Figure II.5), an immunosuppressant used after organ transplantation. The drug functions by reducing interleukine-2 production and is also applicable in the treatment of vitiligo and eczema.

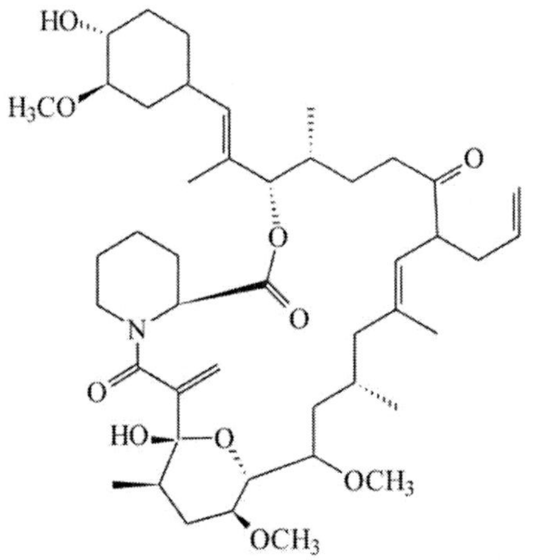

Figure II.5. Tacrolimus, an immunosuppressant drug.

3.3. Bioactive Compounds of Animal Origin

Deer antlers grow rapidly in the spring with the rate of few centimeters each day. This period of intensive cell growth lasts several months. Deer antler velvet has a long history of use in traditional Chinese medicine for treating kidney diseases, strengthening the body and healing chronic wounds. For obvious bioactivity of compounds contained in the antler velvet over the last few decades started a commercial farming of deer to produce antlers. The greatest producers of deer antler velvet are New Zeeland and America. Commercial deer antler velvet products are available in capsule form or as a dry powder. Alcohol extract of deer antlers has been shown to increase phagocytic activity and to modulate immunological response in rats. In addition, proliferation and morphological changes in cultured cell lines of fibroblasts and neuronal cells have been observed under the influence of antler velvet extract and were caused by potent bioactive compounds (Roh et al., 2010). Since rapid rate of antler growth requires rapid angiogenesis it is speculated that bioactive compounds can be used in cancer therapy. This assumption is currently under examination.

3.4. Bioactive Compounds of Marine Origin

Many cases of poisoning by seafood, such as crustaces, fish and mussels, are reported each day worldwide. Human poisoning occurs due to absence of knowledge on the risk that specific marine species carries. Intoxication with marine species is the most difficult to predict because any marine species may represent a potential threat if fed on plankton or sea microorganisms which are frequently a real producers of toxins. In addition to such indirect introduction and carryover, the number of higher marine organisms producing venoms is quite extensive. Due to chemical diversity of potential marine threats, it is difficult to develop a standardized procedure for their detection. Bioaffinity tests are available only for well known and elucidated toxins. Alternative diagnostic tool may include administration of the extract of particular marine organism to experimental mice, however results of such tests are not readily available (Bhakuni and Rawat, 2005).

Tetrodotoxin is a strong neurotoxin produced by different organisms, one of which is a fugu fish. The venom is also produced by terrestrial venomous organisms such as Amazonian poison arrow frogs. The highest concentration of the substance is found in fish ovaries and liver, even though in some fish species the toxin can be well distributed in whole muscle tissue. Meals prepared of fugu may contain low levels of the toxin even after the removal of organs accumulating tetrodotoxin, causing a subtitle tingling in tongue, the feeling the gourmands are seeking for.

The symptoms of tetrodotoxin poisoning start appearing between twenty minutes to three hours upon ingestion and these include vomiting, diarrhea, numbness and tingling in mouth, tongue and lips, and paralysis in conscious state (Švarc-Gajić, 2009). Tetrodotoxin exhibits neurotoxicity by increasing membrane permeability to sodium and blocking the conduction of impulses. Death eventually occurs due to respiratory paralysis.

Saxitoxin, another strong neurotoxin, is produced by mollusk, pufferfish, cyanobacteria (*Aphanizomenon, Anabaena, Lyngbyasp)* and dinoflagellates (*Gymnodinium, Alexandrium, Pyrodinium*). Intoxication with the neurotoxin is known as paralytic shellfish poisoning. Due to some common symptoms, poisoning with saxitoxin can be misdiagnosed with poisoning with other toxins, such as botulinum or tetrodotoxin.

Ciguatoxin is produced by *Gambierdiscus toxicus* algae and is accumulated in tropical and semitropical bottom-feeding fish. Both neural and gastrointestinal symptoms are observed upon poisoning, including nausea, vomiting, parasthesia, numbness and hallucinations (Švarc-Gajić, 2009). The recovery from ciguatera poisoning is very slow and the symptoms may persist for years. The toxin from intoxicated individual can be transmitted sexually and is also excreted in human milk.

4. ISOLATION OF NATURAL BIOACTIVE COMPOUNDS

4.1. Ergot Alkaloids

Ergot alkaloids are produced by artificial infection of cereals with *Claviceps purpurea*. The compounds are unstable, therefore the process of their isolation is complex. Every producer of ergot alkaloids uses different technology. Technological processes are mostly discontinual and of low capacity (10-20 tons/year). At the industrial scale row alkaloids are produced and their further separation and purification is conducted in the laboratory. Quality of produced alkaloids mostly depends on the quality of row material. Parasitic fungus used for the production of ergot alkaloids contains about 30% of fats which causes problems during production, more specifically in the L/L extraction step due to formation of stable emulsions. Prior extractions of alkaloids fats are therefore removed by extraction with petrol ether in which alkaloids are insoluble. After alkali addition, sodium carbonate or magnesium oxide, alkaloids are extracted with ether, benzene, chloroform or dichloroethylene. Purification is performed by adsorption chromatography and crystallization.

During milling step (Figure II.6) the temperature of the mill should be controlled to avoid decomposition of alkaloids. Extraction after alkalinization is performed in the battery of percolators performing multiple extraction stages, and usually up to five steps suffice (Pekić, 1983). The efficiency of the extraction in the battery is usually satisfactory, about 95%. In the battery of average capacity in one extraction cycle up to 150-250 kg of raw material can be extracted. Exhausted raw material is transferred to the destillator (vapor pressure 200-300 kPa) where the solvent residue is removed. Alkaloids are transferred to aqueous solution by L/L extraction with tartaric acid (2:1) performed in multiple stages. In this step emulsion formation may represent a problem. After filtration alkaloids are precipitated by alkali addition. Formed white sediment is separated after 1-2h and is extracted with chloroform. Alkaloids are dried with calcium carbonate and are further transferred to petrol-ether (1:5). Precipitated alkaloids are filtered and further purified. Produced raw alkaloids must be stored in the dark, but before their storage alkaloids are analyzed by spectrophotometry to quantitate individual enantiomers. Individual ergot components are identified by HPLC.

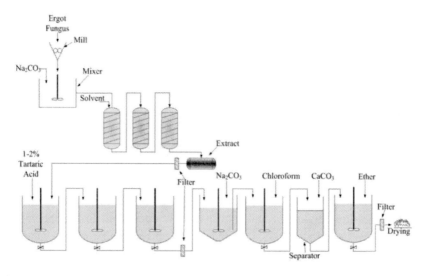

Figure II.6. Industrial production of ergotamine-tartrate.

Produced alkaloids are normally composed of 65-70% of levorotary (-) ergotamine and 30-35% of (+) dextrorotary ergotamine. Since (-) levorotary enantiomer doesn't exhibit physiological activity isomerization is further performed. Raw ergotamine sulfate is precipitated from methanolic solution upon addition of concentrated sulphuric acid (Figure II.7). Sulfates further undergo filtration and dissolution in chloroform saturated with ammonia. Alkaloids are precipitated by adding petrol ether. In precipitate ergotamine represents about 95% (Pekić, 1983). For the removal of other alkaloids water/acetone precristalization is applied. Alkaloids are dissolved in hot acetone and upon water addition alkaloids crystallize. Crystals are filtrated, dried and analyzed for optical activity. Acetone/water precristalization is repeated until sufficient optical purity is achieved. If by repeated precristalization efficient isomerization is not achieved, alkaloids can be again converted to sulphate form. Ergotamine-tartrate is obtained by crystallization from methanolic solution. Crystals of ergotamine are dissolved in hot methanol in 1:20 ratio. After filtration, addition of tartaric acid and cooling, formed white crystals of ergotamine tartrate are separated, washed with methanol and dried under the vacuum. Alkaloid is packed in nitrogen or carbon-dioxide atmospheres in dark bottles because of extreme photosensitivity.

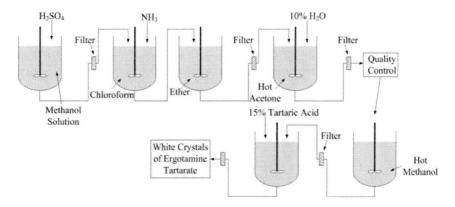

Figure II.7. Isomerization of ergotamine at the industrial scale.

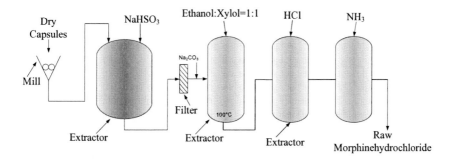

Figure II.8. Industrial production of morphine.

4.2. Opium Alkaloids

Opium alkaloids are produced from dried latex of opium poppy (*Papaver somniferum L.* var. album D.C; *Papaver somniferum L.* var. glabrum Boiss) or dry pods. Raw poppy pods are cut to exude white, milky latex used for the production. Afghanistan and Iran are the largest producers of opium. Dry pods of opium poppy contain approximately 0.2% of opium alkaloids, the most abundant being morphine. In the production process opium or dry, ground capsules are extracted with aqueous solution of $NaHSO_3$ (Figure II.8). The extract is filtered and alkalinized with sodium carbonate, further being extracted with ethanol and xylol (1:1) mixture. Morphine is extracted from the obtained solution with hydrochloric acid and is afterwards precipitated with ammonia.

After morphine extraction other alkaloids that accompany morphine, namely codeine, narcotine, tebain and papaverine, can be separated. Material remaining after morphine extraction is extracted with benzene. Benzene extract is further extracted with 40% NaOH (Figure II.9). Narcotoline, which is high in culinary strains, can be precipitated from the aqueous phase with sulphuric acid (Pekić, 1983). Organic phase is extracted with 50% sulphuric acid. Codeine-sulphate is precipitated and filtrated from the obtained aqueous phase. Joined filtrate and acidic extract obtained after extracting benzene fraction with 5% sulphuric acid, are alkalinized with NaOH precipitating the alkaloids. The precipitate is extracted is dissolved in acetic acid. From the obtained solution tebain is precipitated by the addition of ammonia, whereas insoluble fraction is dissolved in sulphuric acid. By adding ethanolic solution of ammonia narcotine is precipitated. Papaverine is obtained from the filtrate after extraction with benzene and concentration (Pekić, 1983).

4.3. Marine Bioactive Compounds

In the last 25 years, marine organisms, like algae, invertebrates, and microorganisms, have provided key structures and compounds that proved their potential as therapeutic agents for a variety of diseases. The main problem in isolation of bioactive compounds of marine origin is sample collection and taxonomy. Symbiotic communities with bacteria, fungi and microalgae further complicate the task of establishing a source of bioactive compounds. In addition, many marine organisms that produce bioactive compounds are difficult to grow and cultivate.

Some common steps can be recognized in isolation of bioactive principles from marine species. From total methanolic extract of dry raw material the compounds are fractionated according to their polarity (Figure II.10). Aqueous phase, or buthanol fraction, contains alkaloid salts, aminoacids, polyhydroxysteroids and other polar compounds. Medium polarity compounds, like peptides and depsipeptides, can be separated by dichloromethanol, whereas hexane and carbon tetrachloride are good solvents for low polarity molecules, such as hydrocarbons, fatty acids, acetogenins and terpens. After separating compounds to polarity classes, all fractions are tested

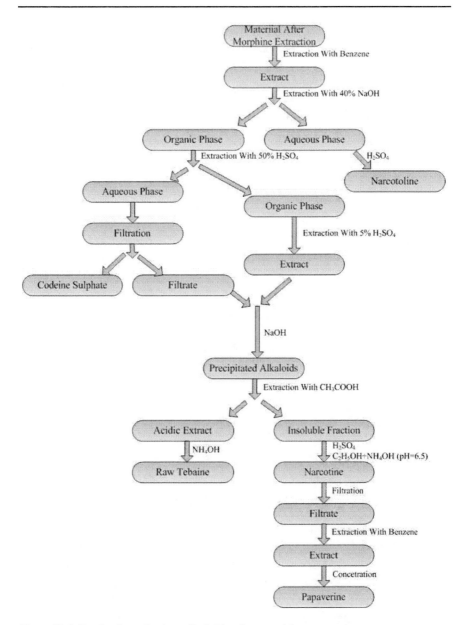

Figure II. 9. Production of opium alkaloids after morphine removal.

for bioactivity. Fraction in which bioactivity was detected is further separated to individual compounds by preparative chromatography and HPLC to detect individual compounds. From the polar fraction chlorides and other minerals must be removed by ion-exchange resin (Amberlite) or size exclusion (Sephadex) chromatography (Riguera, 1997). Active aqueous fraction is further separated to individual compounds by countercurrent chromatography or HPLC.

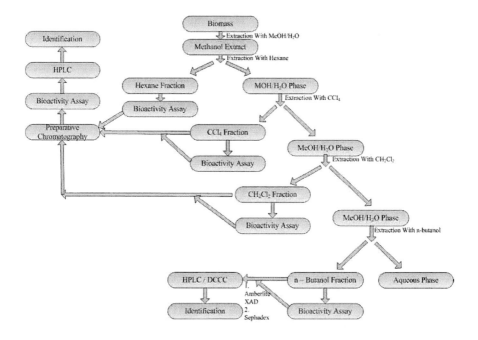

Figure II.10. Fractionation of bioactive compounds from marine organisms.

After individual components have been isolated in their pure form, they must by identified by using combination of different spectroscopic techniques. When applying mass spectrometry soft ionization techniques, such as chemical ionization, FAB, thermospray or electrospray ionization must be applied in order to prevent abundant molecular defragmentation. Identification of individual molecular parts, units and fragments, for complex molecules composed of several units, such as peptides, oligosaccharides or saponins, is performed by tandem mass spectrometry.

REFERENCES

Bhakuni DS and Rawat DS. *Bioactive marine organisms*. Springer, New York, 2005.

Ernst E. A systematic review of systematic reviews of homeopathy. *British J Clin Pharm* 54 (6), 2002, 577–582.

Leistner E and Drewke C. *Ginkgo biloba* and Ginkgotoxin. *J Na Prod*.73 (1), 2010, 86–92.

Pekić B. Hemija i tehnologija farmaceutskih proizvoda (alklaoidi i etarska ulja). *Tehnološki fakultet,* Novi Sad, 1983.

Riguera R. Isolating bioactive compounds from marine organisms. *J Mar Biotech* 5, 1997, 187-193.

Roh SS, Lee MH, Hwang YL, Song HH, Jin MH, Park SG, Lee CK, Kim CD, Yoon TJ, Lee JH. Stimulation of the extracellular matrix production in dermal fibroblasts by velvet antler extract. *Ann Derm.* 22(2), 2010,173-179.

Švarc-Gajić J. Naturally occurring food toxicants. In: *Nutritional insights in food safety* (Ed: Švarc-Gajić J. Nova Science Publishers, New York, 2011), 39-99.

Chapter III

MEDICINAL USE OF SOME PHYTOCHEMICALS

Up to date more than 10 000 phytochemicals have been identified. Phytochemicals refer to non-nutritive, non-essential and bioactive plant chemicals. Throughout the history numerous beneficial effects of phytochemicals have been recognized. For some compounds it is known that they protect cells against oxidative damage and reduce the risk of developing certain types of cancer. Phytoestrogens may help to reduce menopausal symptoms and osteoporosis. Many of compounds from this class act as enzyme inductors or inhibitors. Diterpenes from coffee and vegetable indoles can activate microsomal enzymes, whereas grapefruit must be avoided when taking drug therapy due to presence of strong inhibitors bergamottin and paradisine. Some phytochemicals act physically, such as proanthocyanidins from cranberries that bind to cell walls of the urinary tract preventing the adhesion of pathogens to human cell walls.

In 19th and 20th centuries many bioactive compounds have been discovered, such as salicylic acid, morphine and pyrethroids. Developments of analytical techniques introduced an improvement in identification of new phytochemicals, making it more reliable. With the development of organic synthesis discovered and identified compounds were able to be synthetized. Modern approach to phytochemistry implies exploitation of bioengineering techniques to increase natural production in plants.

1. KAVA-KAVA

Kava-kava is a pungent crop grown in the Pacific. The plant is traditionally used in Polynesia, Micronesia, Melanesia and other Pacific regions to prepare beverage for treating insomnia, stress and anxiety, or for consumption during ceremonial occasions such as weddings. The beverage is prepared from dried, powdered roots with the addition of lecithin which acts like an emulsifier and helps water extraction. Due to high pharmacological activity kava-kava is listed in the Pharmacopeia of Oceania and in 1914 kava was listed in the British Pharmacopoeia.

In traditional medicine kava is used for different purposes. Kava extracts applied topically are used to treat fungal infections, stings and skin inflammations. Antibacterial effects of kava are very strong and this is supported by the fact that in kava-drinking population low incidence of gonorrhea is reported. Kava beverages provoke sedation, talkative and euphoric behavior in consumers. Experienced tongue numbing is caused by local constriction of blood vessels (Švarc-Gajić, 2011). Anesthetic potency of kava bioactive compounds is believed to be close to that of cocaine, whereas its analgetic effect is stronger of that of aspirin. In traditional medicine kava was used as anticonvulsant because it was established that it enhances control over grand mal.

Bioactive compounds of kava-kava are known as kava lactones and have been a subject of research since 1800s. As many as fifteen kava lactones are known, but only seven appear in kava to significant extent. Dihydromethysticin is recognized as the most active tranquilizer of all kava lactones. Dihydrokawain is produced during aging of the roots. Fresh roots contain only 0.2% of dihydrokawain, whereas the roots dried for one year contains up to 1% and older roots may contain up to 3% of the substance (Švarc-Gajić, 2011). Kava lactones were also isolated from a plant grown in Japan, *Alpinia speciosa*.

Side effects of consuming kava beverage include headache, visual disturbances and strong diuresis. Allergic reactions and disturbance of clotting processes may also be demonstrated. On the basis of animal studies it was estimated that for humans up to 1-2 kg of kava root is safe. Concerns about kava safety have been raised primarily in respect to chronic kava consumption, due to observed kidney and liver damage in kava consumers. Observed adverse effects, however, could not been linked to sole kava-kava influence and are possibly related to the influence of other substances, such as alcohol or drugs, or to preexisting liver pathology. Another speculation is that in persons in which liver damage was observed, beverage was not prepared from plants roots, but other plant parts containing toxic substances. A toxic alkaloid pipermethystine, isolated from stem peelings and leaves, demonstrated hepatotoxicity in both *in vitro* and *in vivo* trials. Flavokavain B (Figure III.1) is another toxic principle that was found in plant's rhizome (Teschke et al., 2011).

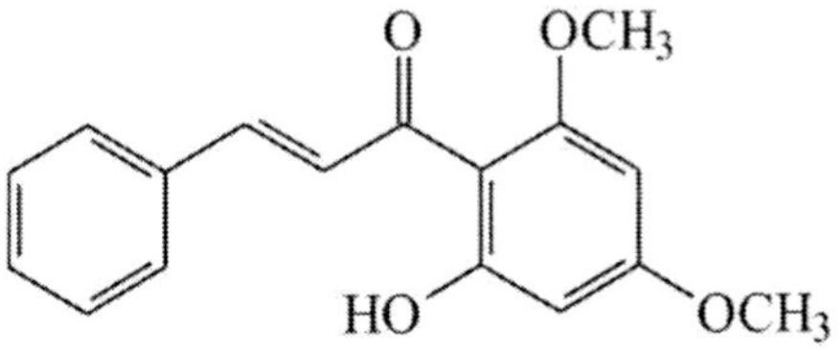

Figure III.1. Flavokavain B.

2. PHENYLALANINE

Phenylalanine is essential amino acid which is converted to important catecholamines in the brain. Amino acid is converted to L-dopa, epinephrine, norepinephrine, as well as to some thyroid hormones via tyrosine. Because norepinephrine affects mood, different forms of phenylalanine preparations have been proposed to treat depression. Chemically similar to amphetamine, phenylethylamine is a mild alkaloid stimulant produced naturally in the body as a by-product of phenylalanine. In metabolic disorder called phenylketonuria phenylalanine is not properly metabolized causing its build-up. The condition is diagnosed in the first 48 - 72 hours of life. Untreated phenylketonuria can cause severe and irreversible mental retardation. People with phenylketonuria must avoid phenylalanine and take must regularly take tyrosine supplements.

Animal sources of phenylalanine include meat, fish, milk, yogurt, eggs and cheese. Aspartame is a methyl ester of phenylalanine dipeptide. Nuts, lima beans, pumpkin and sesame seeds and various soy products are rich plant sources of phenylalanine. Of two phenylalanine enantiomers which demonstrate different biological effects, D is not present in natural products, but is made artificially. Analgetic effects are attributed to D-phenylalanine, which blocks enkephalinase which degrades enkephalins, naturally occurring substances that reduce pain. L-phenylalanine supplements due to their implication in brain chemistry are used by patients with Parkinsonism and schizophrenia (Walsh et al., 1986; Talkowski et al., 2009). This enantiomer is also able to initiate repigmentation of the skin and is used to treat vitiligo. The use of phenylalanine supplements must not be combined with the use of anti-depressants such as MAO inhibitors and must be avoided in pregnancy. Individuals with heart problems and malignant melanomas should also avoid these dietary supplements.

3. PHYTOESTROGENS

Phytoestrogens are naturally occurring non-steroidal compounds which have been identified in more than 300 plant species. Their bioactivity arises from mimicking biochemical effects of estrogen. Phytoestrogens act as agonists or antagonists of 17-β-estradiol. Flax seed and soybeans have been identified as food containing among the highest levels of phytoestrogens.

Flavones, Isoflavones, lignans and coumestans are major classes of phytoestrogens. Isoflavones are found in high concentration in soy products, whereas in flax seed lignans are predominant. Coumestans are found in peas, beans and alfalfa. This class of phytoestrogens is least studied even though it has the strongest interaction with receptors and estrogen-like effects.

Phytoestrogens can act like estrogen at low doses but on the other hand may block estrogen at high concentrations. Estrogen replacement affects the production of estrogen by the body. This may affect communication pathways between cells and prevent the formation of blood vessels, contributing to tumor formation. Furthermore, the changes in the form of estrogen which in excess circulates through the system may cause cell mutation. The effects of circulating estrogen forms in different parts of the body may be different.

Conducted studies on the relationship between breast cancer and soy in the diet are not straightforward. Animal studies suggest that soy phytoestrogens under certain circumstances can behave like estrogen and may potentially increase breast cancer risk (Švarc-Gajić, 2011). Risk in humans, however, in general is not so serious because food rich in phytoestrogens usually represents only small portion of the diet, and phytoestrogens have several times less potent biochemical activity in comparison to estrogen hormones. Soy-based infant formulas have the highest levels of phytoestrogens and it is estimated that babies whose diet is based on such formulations are exposed to ten times greater concentrations of phytoestrogens than adult vegetarians (Tuohy, 2003).

Feed rich in phytoestrogen-producing plants may negatively influence the reproduction in grazing animals and may contribute to infertility in livestock. Genistein and coumestrol, found in feed, deposit in fat tissue of animals and may provoke uterine hypertrophy and alter mammary gland differentiation.

4. PSORALENS

Psoralens or furocoumarins are synthetized by plants as protective agents against wide range of threats, from insects to mammals. In these phototoxic compounds furan ring is fused to coumarin. The compounds are found in celery, lime, fig, bergamot, lemon, fennel, parsnip, carrot, as well as in numerous pasture plants like *Tribulus terrestris*, *Pannicum laevifolium*, *Pannicum coloratum* and *Fagopyrum cymosum*. The content of psoralens in vegetables increases with aging and is higher in old and damaged plants.

After handling or consumption of psoralene-producing plants and subsequent exposure to sunlight, severe phototoxic reactions mat develop. Topical contact with plants containing psoralens has been shown to represent more serious risk to skin damage in comparison to ingestion of such food. In addition to local reactions, ingestion of psoralene-rich foods, such as celery, can cause generalized phototoxicity. Developed phytophotodermatitis closely resembles contact dermatitis or chemical burns, and progresses further to post-inflammatory hyperpigmentation. The rash typically appears 36 to 72 h after exposure and lasts for one to two weeks. Postinflammatory hyperpigmentation can persist for weeks or months. In grazing animals affected skin turns brown and hard and conjunctiva and mucosa membrane in mouth become yellow (Švarc-Gajić, 2011). Animals become photosensitive. Due to skin damaging properties in prolonged exposures psoralens may contribute to cancer formation. Skin burns and blisters provoked by psoralens and UV light are treated topically or systemically by corticosteroids.

In the treatment of skin depigmentation psoralens have been used for centuries. Today the compounds are used as phototherapeutic agents to treat cutaneous lymphoma, psoriasis and vitiligo. The compounds alter the activity of microsomal enzymes, thus influencing metabolic biotransformation of natural substances as well as xenobiotics. For this reason it is not recommended to take grapefruit during drug therapy, because it is high in bergamottin (Figure III.2) and dihydroxybergamottin, characteristic psoralens.

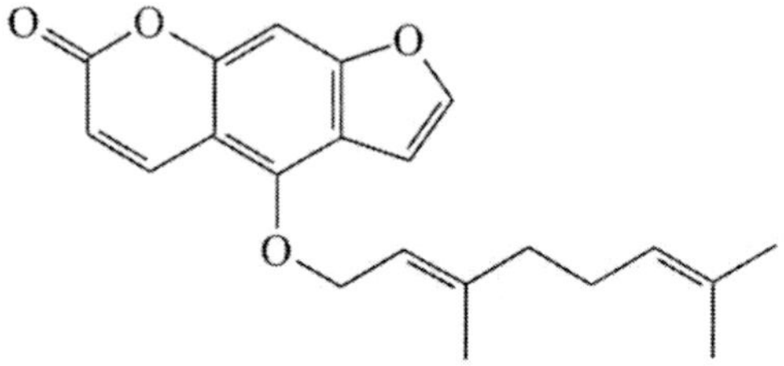

Figure III.2. Bergamottin – a psoralene isolated from grapefruit.

As phototherapeutic agents psoralens are available in pill, lotions and bath salts form. They are used to treat severe psoriasis in which more than 20% of the body is affected. Psoralens are administrated to patients 2h before exposure to UV light 2-3 times per week. The concentration of psoralens is usually not changed but rather the intensity of the light (Serrano-Perez et al., 2008). Phototherapy with psoralens has numerous side effects, such as increased risk of a skin cancer, skin redness and itching, skin keratosis and spread of psoriasis to skin areas that were not affected before. Male genitals are highly susceptible to cancer-inducing effects, whereas female genitals do not seem to be affected (Serrano-Perez et al., 2008).

5. SAFROLE

Sassafras species (*Sassafras albidum, Sassafras hesperia, Sassafras randaiense*) are medium-sized, aromatic trees, native to USA, Canada and Mexico. The root bark of sassafras is used for the production of aromatic oil by steam distillation. The principal compound responsible for its characteristic fragrance is *safrole* (Figure III.3). Safrole is also present in myriad of other plant species, such as cinnamon, nutmeg, pepper, basil, wormseed, Japanese star anise and others, but sassafras are particularly high in safrole. The compound constitutes up to 80% of the root bark oil.

Due to its distinctive flavor sassafras have long been used culinary. Dried and ground sassafras leaves were used as a spice for preparing specific types of stews. The leaves can be used in salads. Young shoots were used to make characteristic American root bear, but today sassafras food products have been withdrawn by authority agencies due to recognized adverse health effects.

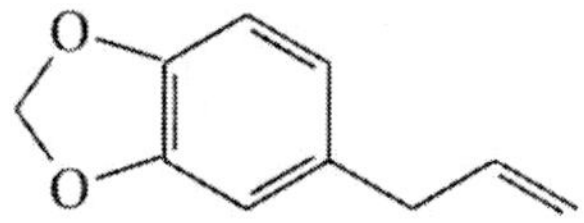

Figure III.3. Safrole.

In traditional medicine sassafras in the form of powder, oil, extracts and tinctures, are still used for various health conditions. Sassafras oil is used as a fungicide and to treat gonorrhea. Dried bark in doses of 10 g is used as carminative.

Fatal toxicity in sassafras oil consumption has been reported primarily due to sassafras abuse. Namely, safrole is a precursor to amphetamine, which is responsible for effects in central nervous system, such as increased self-awareness, empathy, communicativeness, and euphoria. Searching for such effects, sassafras abusers were acutely intoxicated demonstrating vomiting, stupor and hallucinations.

Safrole and isosafrole (4-propenyl-1,2-methylenedioxybenzene), it's naturally occurring isomer, according to conducted animals studies, form DNA adducts with guanine provoking liver tumors (Švarc-Gajić, 2011). In liver they are dealkylated followed by electron transfer, oxidation to o-quinone and isomerization to p-quinone. In addition to being hepatotoxic they induce hepatic microsomal enzymes cytochrome P-488, cytochrome P-450 and biphenyl hydroxylase.

6. SEROTONIN

Serotonin is a monoamine neurotransmitter biochemically derived from tryptophan via 5-HTP (L-5-hydroxytryphtophan) (Figure III.4). The compound regulates mood, appetite, sleep and is involved in memory and learning. Serotonin receptors are found in gastrointestinal tract, platelets and central nervous system. In the gut, serotonin regulates intestinal movements. Plants are able to synthesize serotonin and this bioactive compound is relatively high in bananas, plantains, aubergine, pineapple, avocado, walnuts and plums.

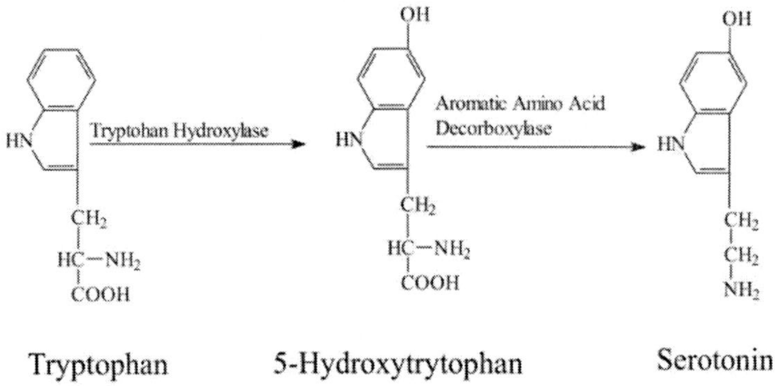

Tryptophan   5-Hydroxytrytophan   Serotonin

Figure III.4. The production of serotonin in the body.

Serotonin metabolite, 5-hydroxyindoleacetic acid (Figure III.5), is excreted in urine and is monitored to determine the body's levels of serotonin. Serotonin overproduction occurs in cancer and values greater than 25 mg of serotonin in urine per 24 hours indicate cancerous process (Schultz, 1987). Diagnosis, however, may be influenced by different pathological conditions. Patients with renal diseases may have falsely low 5-hydroxyindoleacetic acid levels, whereas in patients with celiac disease, cystic fibrosis and chronic intestinal obstruction the levels can be falsely elevated.

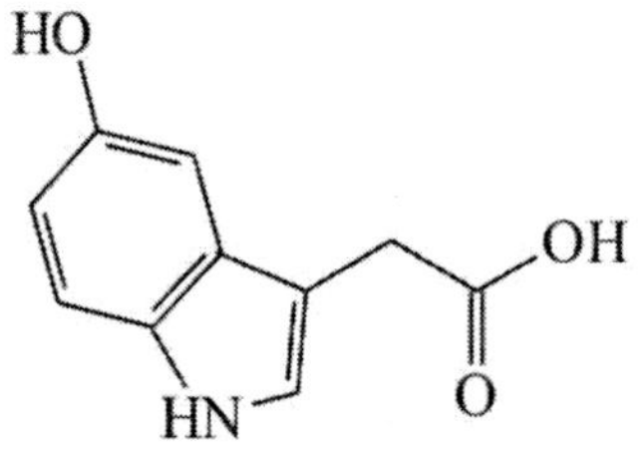

Figure III.5. 5-Hydroxyindoleacetic acid, a serotonin metabolite.

Serotonin supplements are used in the treatment of Alzheimer's, anxiety, depression, headaches and memory loss.

7. CAROTENOIDS

Carotenoids are produced by plants, microorganisms and marine organisms representing yellow, red and orange pigments. Among more than 600 known carotenoids only 50 of them demonstrate pro-vitamin activity. Vitamin activity of beta-carotene, a precursor of vitamin A, is approximately one twelfth of that of retinol. Carotenoids can be classified to xanthophylls containing oxygen, and carotenes which are purely hydrocarbons. In plants and algeae the pigments absorb light energy for use in photosynthesis, and they protect chlorophyll from photodamage. In addition to pro-vitamin A activity carotenoids demonstrate other effects in the body, such as antioxidant, light filtering and influence on intercellular communication via stimulation of cell membranes protein synthesis.

Lutein and zeaxanthin, two stereoisomers, belong to xanthophylls group. Deposited in eyes they absorb blue light reducing light-induced oxidative damage. Meso-zeaxanthin is a third discovered xanthophyll formed in the retina from lutein. The pigments are found in green leafy vegetables, fruits, corn and egg yolk. In green vegetables the color of pigments is often masked with chlorophyll. Being highly lipophylic lutein and zeaxanthin require the presence of dietary fat for good absorption through digestive tract. These xanthophylls are also deposited in small quantities in the skin, contributing to its color, as well as in the blood, brain and breast.

Adverse effects of these pigments rarely occur as a consequence of dietary intake, but rather through elevated supplements intake. At elevated concentrations breathing problems, chest pain, dizziness and irritation in eyes and skin may be experienced (Harikumar et al., 2008).

Lycopene is a bright red pigment belonging to a carotene class. Among all carotenoids lycopene is one of the most effective quenchers of singlet oxygen radicals. Chemically it is tetraterpenoid composed of eight isoprene units (Figure III.6). While not exhibiting pro-vitamin activity, lycopene demonstrates strong antioxidant effects due to conjugated double bonds.

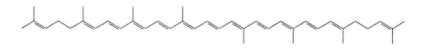

Figure III.6. Lycopene.

Lycopene is an important intermediate in biosynthesis of other carotenoids. Among 72 possible geometric isomers cis forms have the bent form, whereas $trans$ are linear molecules. Bioactivity among isomers may vary significantly, and is virtually impossible to be determined due to unavailability of individual standard isomers.

Lycopene is high in red and orange fruits and vegetables. Pigment is also abundant in salmon, shellfish and milk, and particularly high in gac, a fruit native to south Asia, where it reaches the contents up to 2000 µg/g of wet weight. Food processing increases lycopene bioavailability, releasing it from its complexes with fibers and other food components. Since lycopene is very unpolar molecule in order to be absorbed from the gastrointestinal tract, the presence of dietary fat is required. In this way lycopene dissolves in fat droplets subsequently forming micelles with bile salts, which are able to penetrate to intestinal mucosal cells by passive diffusion (Figure III.7).

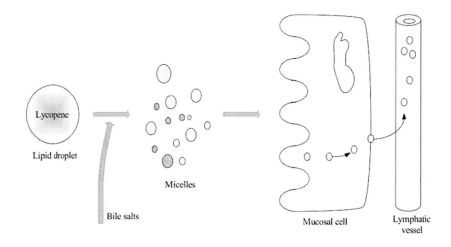

Figure III.7. Absorption of lycopene from the gastrointestinal tract.

Lycopene exhibits potent antioxidant capacity with quenching ability hundred times higher than vitamin E, as well as other effects (Kong and Ismail, 2011). This pigment efficiently reduces skin damage caused by UV light and acts as an activator of phase II enzymes.

Health risks associated to high lycopene intake are linked to lycopene producing itself reactive radicals in the body, especially when taken in supplement form and under the influence of external factors, such as cigarette smoke. In this instance lycopene may act as a carcinogen. Lycopene is available in supplement form individually or mixed with other carotenoids in oil-based formulations.

REFERENCES

Harikumar KB, Nimita CV, Preethi KC, Kuttan R, Shankaranarayana ML, Deshpande J. Toxicity profile of lutein and lutein ester isolated from marigold flowers (*Tagetes erecta*). *Int J Tox*. 27(1), 2008,1-9.

Kong KW and Ismail A. Lycopene content and lipophilic antioxidant capacity of by-products from *Psidium guajava* fruits produced during puree production industry. *Food Bio Proc* 89(1), 2011, 53–61.

Schultz AL. 5-Hydroxyindoleacetic Acid. In: *Methods in Clinical Chemistry* (Eds: Pesce AJ and Kaplan LA).Mosby-Year Book Inc., 1987, 714-720.

Serrano-Perez JJ, Serrano-Andres L, Merchan M. Photosensitization and phototherapy with furocoumarins: A quantum-chemical study. *Chem Physics* 347, 2008, 422–435.

Švarc-Gajić J. Naturally occurring food toxicants. In: *Nutritional insights in food safety* (Ed: Švarc-Gajić J. Novascience Publishers, New York, 2011), 39-99.

Talkowski ME, McClain L, Allen T, Bradford LD, Calkins M, Edwards N, Georgieva L, Go R, Gur R, Gur R, Kirov G, Chowdari K, Kwentus J, Lyons P, Mansour H, McEvoy J, O'Donovan MC, O'Jile J, Owen MJ, Santos A, Savage R, Toncheva D, Vockley G, Wood J, Devlin B, Nimgaonkar VL. Convergent patterns of association between phenylalanine hydroxylase variants and schizophrenia in four independent samples. *Am J Med Genet B Neur Gen*. 150 B(4), 2009, 560-569.

Teschke R, Qiu SX, Lebot V. Herbal hepatotoxicity by kava: update on pipermethystine, flavokavain B, and mould hepatotoxins as primarily assumed culprits. *Dig Liver Dis*. 43(9), 2011, 676-681.

Tuohy PG. Soy infant formula and phytoestrogens. *J Paediatr Child Health*. 39(6), 2003, 401-405

Walsh NE, Ramamurthy S, Schoenfeld L, Hoffman J. Analgesic effectiveness of D-phenylalanine in chronic pain patients. *Arch Phys Med Rehabil*. 67(7), 1986, 436-439.

Chapter IV

MEDICINAL USE OF ALKALOIDS

Alkaloids represent medicinally very important class of compounds, synthetized by plants, insects, marine organisms, mammals and microorganisms. This class of compounds was first discovered in plants for what they were denoted as plant alkalis. It is estimated that they are synthetized by 10 -15% of the plants. Majority of alkaloids are crystalline, colorless substances, even though liquid alkaloids, like nicotine, also exist. Some of alkaloids are colored, like berberine. Alkaloids are more stable when are in the salt form.

Being secondary metabolites alkaloids are formed from proteins and are considered to be of the highest toxicity to predators and man, among other naturally occurring compounds. Chemically, majority of natural alkaloids are heterocyclic, with the exception of protoalkaloids, like mescaline, ephedrine and hordenine, which have nitrogen in a side chain. Alkaloids encompass very broad spectrum of chemically diverse compounds and their classification is very complex. Several criteria can be applied to divide them to classes, e.g. according to biological activity, according to producing species, or according to ring system containing nitrogen atom.

1. ERGOT ALKALOIDS

Ergot alkaloids belong to indole class and are produced by *Claviceps purpurea,* a parasitic fungus that grows on rye and other cereals. Poisoning with ergot alkaloids strike Europe severely in the Middle Ages. Between 6th and 18th century 132 epidemics of ergotism were reported in Europe.

Symptomatology of ergotism dependents on the dominant type of present alkaloids. In convulsive ergotism nervous system is mostly affected, whereas in gangrenous ergotism blood vessels are damaged. In the past gangrenous ergotism was known as St. Anthony's Fire due to burning sensation in extremities that was provoked by damaged blood vessels.

Far back in the history it was observed that grazing on grass infected with ergot alkaloids caused the abortion in pregnant farm animals. The first bioactive effect that was linked to ergot was the ability to induce smooth muscle contractions. In traditional medicine the fungus was adopted as oxytocic to perform abortions and to accelerate uterine contractions of women in labor. Since dosage could not be given accurately due to large variations in active ingredients, as well as due to numerous side effects, such as violent nausea, vomiting and uterine rupture, ergot was abandoned as oxytocic drug. It was only during the 20th century that ergot was shown to be useful in the treatment of migraine attacks.

For its potent bioactivity today the fungus is artificially parasitically cultivated by infecting the crops or by *in vitro* cultivation. Fungal sclerotium has high oil content (30-40%) making the extraction of alkaloids quite difficult. Besides alkaloids fungus also produces numerous other biologically active substances, such as acetylcholine, histamine, tyramine, ergosterin, uracil, betaine and others.

Ergot alkaloids affect alpha-adrenergic, dopamine and serotonin receptors inducing constriction of smooth muscles and walls of small blood vessels (Rowell and Larson, 1999). Damage to blood vessels is often irreversible. Gangrenous ergotism first starts with tingling, numbness and feeling of cold in fingers and toes, followed by gangrene progression in limbs and in some cases complete loss of limbs (De Costa, 2002). In convulsive ergotism hallucinations, delirium and epileptic-type seizures are observed (Eadie, 2003). In the Middle Ages people with convulsive ergotism were considered to be affected by witchcraft. In intoxicated persons pupils are first contracted but in later stages they dilate. Neurological symptoms may sustain even after the alkaloids have been excreted.

Chemically, ergot alkaloids may be divided to *clavinet type* and *lysergic acid amides*. Natural amides of lysergic acid can further be divided into *water soluble* and *water insoluble*. Water insoluble derivatives of lysergic acid contain at least three amino acids in a peptide moiety, whereas in water soluble derivatives lysergic acid or its isomer is bound to an amino alcohol. Clavinet type ergot alkaloids (Figure IV.1) have been also isolated from higher plants and are precursors in biosynthesis of other ergot alkaloids. They demonstrate powerful uterine stimulation and inhibition of prolactin release. Prolactin is important peptide hormone involved in lactation, immune regulation, angiogenesis and blood clotting.

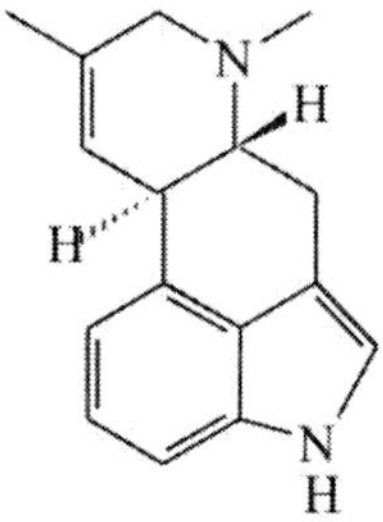

Agroclavine 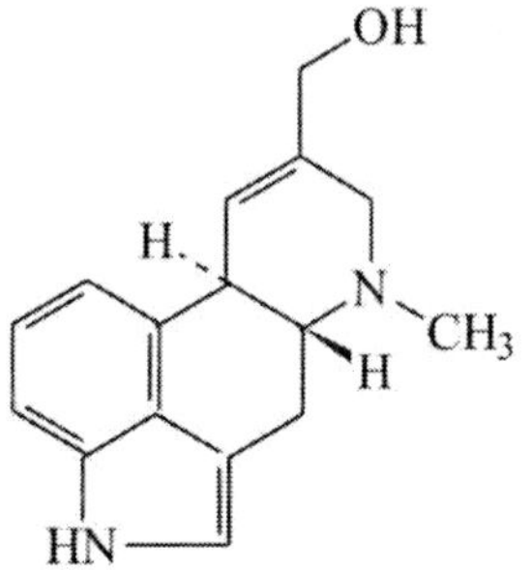   Elymoclavine

Figure IV.1. Clavinet type ergot alkaloids.

Ergonovine is water soluble amide of lysergic acid which provokes strong uterine contractions and has been used through history as a mean of abortion. *Methysergide*, a semisynthetic alkaloid belonging to the same class, is pharmacologically used to treat severe migraines due to its specific vasodilatating properties in cranial brain regions. Methysergide acts like serotonin antagonist, dilating the vessels around the brain, thereby relieving the migraine and headache symptoms (Gallo et al., 1975). The drug is used mostly in prophylaxis of migraines. *Ergotamine* (Figure IV.2), on the other hand, is used in the treatment of acute migraines. The alkaloid belongs to water insoluble group. Antimigraine effects of the compound are, as in the case of methysergide, mediated by neural and vascular serotonin receptors. On oppose to methysergide the alkaloid acts like serotonin agonist producing vasoconstriction. Ergotamine also activates dopamine and epinephrine receptors and is used in the treatment of cerebrovascular insufficiency and Parkinsonism. In ergotamine therapy side effect like tingling, contraction of the uterus, drowsiness and dizziness may be observed.

After oral administration ergotamine follows extensive first-pass effect making its bioavailability extremely low (<1%) for what it is administrated mostly in the form of suppositoria. The compound is mostly excreted in bile. Plasma half-life is 2h and its effects may last up to 24h (Sanders et al., 1986).

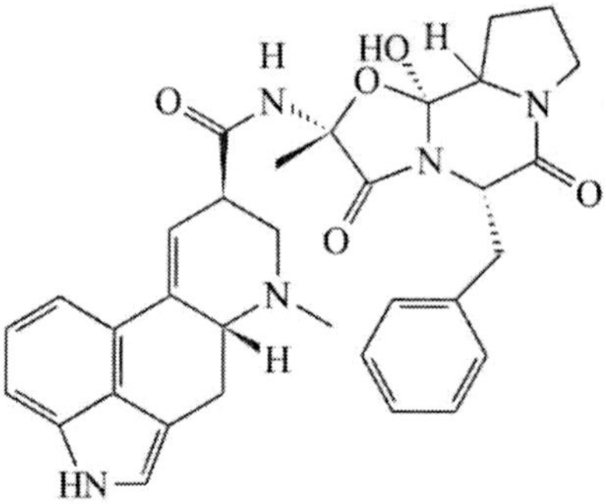

Figure IV.2. Ergotamine.

Ergocryptine is water insoluble amide which can conveniently be used in LSD synthesis rather than ergotamine. In modern medicine mostly semisynthetic brom-ergocryptine is used to treat the absence of a menstrual period in a women of reproductive age and Parkinsonism (Samuelsson, 1999).

Ergometrine (Figure IV.3) is a water soluble amide of lysergic acid. Medically it is used with oxytocin to facilitate delivery of placenta after childbirth. Alkaloid acts via alpha-adrenergic, dopaminergic and serotonin receptors. Ergometrine has also found its application in medical diagnosis, because it is able to induce spasm of the coronary arteries for what it is used to diagnose angina. Ergometrine may provoke LSD-like effects but at dosages much higher than the clinical ones (2–10 mg).

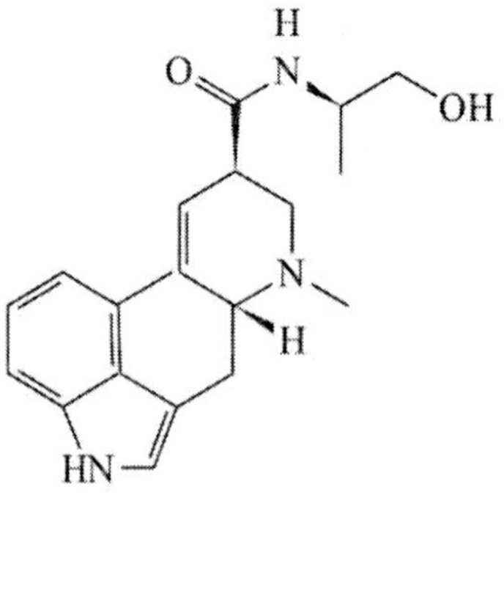

Figure IV.3. Ergometrine.

Overdose of egometrine produces prolonged vasospasm resulting in permanent damage to blood vessels and gangrene development, hallucinations and possible abortions, for what it is contraindicated in pregnancy, vascular diseases and psychosis. Prolonged use of ergometrine decreases oxygen delivery to tissues due to constricted blood vessels.

LSD or lysergic acid diethylamide is semisynthetic derivative that was first synthetized in 1938 by Albert Hofmann and is known for its hallucinogenic properties. Hofmann described hallucinogenic properties after testing it personally. The compound is already active at very low doses interacting with different subtypes of dopamine and serotonin receptors, for what it was extensively used as a tool for elucidating biochemically the behavior. Some individuals who have used LSD experienced persistent perceptual abnormalities which lasted for weeks or months after last exposure (Halpern and Harrison, 2003). Alkaloid was proposed in the treatment of psychosis, however due to its pronounced side effects the idea was abandoned.

All ergot alkaloids are contraindicated in persons undergoing therapy with drugs that affect serotonin, such as Fluoxetine (Prozac) or Paroxetine (Paxil). These are used to treat different neurological disorders, like depression, bipolar disorder, obsessive compulsive disorder, bulimia nervosa, panic disorder and others.

2. PURINE ALKALOIDS

Purine alkaloids are also called xantines and belong to indole group. These pseudoalkaloids are abundantly found in tea plant, coffee and cocoa and are not biosynthesized from amino acids like majority of alkaloids. Representatives, caffeine, theophylline and theobromine, differ only in position of methyl groups. Although abundantly found in plants, theophyllineis now produced synthetically for its medicinal use as a smooth muscle relaxant in the treatment of bronchial asthma. In tea the doses of theophylline are much lower than therapeutic ones.

Caffeine, or 1,3,7-trimethylxanthin, is a water-soluble xantines alkaloid found in coffee, guarana, yerba mate and other plants, where it plays a role of a natural insecticide. At moderate doses caffeine is not toxic to humans, however in animals such as dogs and horses even moderate doses might provoke intoxication. It is considered that caffeine in small doses is beneficial for heart function since glycolysis and ATP production in heart muscle cells enhance after binding of caffeine to receptors on the surface of heart muscle cells (Chapman and Miller, 1974). In addition, caffeine affects respiratory and vasomotor centers of the brain and induces fatty acid metabolism.

Moderate doses of caffeine decrease fatigue and give the feeling of alertness. Acute overdose is accompanied with panic attacks, seizures, tremors and different forms of phobia. Chronic ingestion of high doses of caffeine may induce bone porosity, insomnia, anxiety and psychomotor agitation.

Theophylline is 1,3-dimethylxanthin and was first extracted from tea leaves and chemically identified around 1888 by German biologist Albrecht Kossel. After isolation it was soon synthetized. In medical practice theophylline was first used as diuretic and only much later it started to be used in asthma treatment.

The principal mechanism of theophylline toxicity arises from the excess of adrenalin and noradrenalin which are released after theophylline binding to adrenergic β1 and β2 receptors (Emerman et al., 1990). Theophylline increases blood pressure by affecting heart muscle contractility and has anti-inflammatory effect. After absorption theophylline is metabolized by cytochrome P450 via N-demethylation following first order kinetics. As other xantine alkaloids it is able to pass placental and blood/brain barrier. Moderate toxicity of theophylline, accompanied with irritability, nausea, arrhythmia and tachycardia, is potentiated with erythromycin and cimetidine. Medicinally theophylline is used in the treatment of asthma, other pulmonary diseases and apnea, whereas its effects on the sense of smell are currently under investigation.

Theobromine or 3,7-dimethylxanthine, is found in cocoa, acai berries, cola nuts, tea and other plants. The alkaloid exhibits stimulating properties similar to caffeine, but about ten times weaker. The substance is not very toxic in humans, but in animals like dogs, horses, cats and parrots, it can induce seizures, heart attack and internal bleeding.

3. NUX-VOMICA ALKALOIDS

Nux-Vomica alkaloids are produced by *Strychnos Nux-vomica*, a small tree widely distributed in India, Sri Lanka, Thailand and Northern Australia. The fruit of the plant resembles orange with seeds usually containing about 2-3% of the powerful poisonous alkaloids strychnine and brucine. Strychnine is several times more toxic than brucine. In different parts of the plant hemitoxiferine, a degradation product of strychnine, as well as loganin, a biosynthetic precursor of strychnine, can be found.

In the 17th century the seeds of Strychnos seeds were intensively used in Europe as rodenticide to kill dogs, cats, and birds. The major active principle of the seeds was identified in 1818, and the compound was later on synthetized by Robert B. Woodward. This was considered to be one of the most famous syntheses in the history of organic chemistry. Due to very potent pharmacological activity, pure strychnine is nowadays intensively produced, with India being a major exporter of Strychnos seeds.

Strychnine acts as extremely strong neurotoxin affecting motor nerves in the spinal cord which control muscle contraction. An alkaloid acts as antagonist to glycine and acetylcholine (Miyakawa et al., 2002). Glycine has specific role in CNS acting as an inhibitor of neurons in the brain and the spinal cord. By antagonizing glycine motor neurons are continually being stimulated under the influence of strychnine.

After absorption strychnine binds moderately to plasma proteins being also available in its free form for distribution to other tissues. Strychnine is mostly distributed to liver, kidneys and stomach wall (Gupta, 2009). Within few minutes after ingestion the compound can be detected in urine mostly unchanged.

Symptoms of poisoning with strychnine usually appear within 15 to 60 minutes with nervousness, restlessness and twitching. As poisoning progresses, muscular twitching becomes more pronounced and it proceeds with seizures (Sharma, 2008). As death approaches, convulsions follow one another with increased rapidity, severity and duration. In fatal intoxications death may occur after two hours, but in some cases the outcome can be delayed for six hours. Lethal outcome usually results from respiratory failure due to overstimulation of muscles of the respiratory tract.

In strychnine poisoning there is no antidote available. It is necessary to remove the substance from the system by gastric lavage, emesis or activated charcoal. In order to oxidize any unabsorbed strychnine permanganate or tannins may be administrated. In poisoning with strychnine it is important to administrate strong vasodilatator, such as amyl nitrite and to inhale chloroform in order to alleviate breathing. To restrain seizures and spasms phenobarbital, diazepam and chloral may be useful. Intoxicated individuals must be held in quiet and dark because even the slightest air current or a light beam may trigger the seizures.

Brucine is less toxic than strychnine and does not provoke convulsions and spasms. It inactivates minor motor nerves, for what it may be used as a local analgesic in the treatment of itching.

In traditional Chinese medicine, as well as in homeopathy, Strychnos seeds have very important place. In order to reduce their toxicity the seeds are dried in the sun or are heated. In Unani medicine the seeds are detoxified by holding them in water for 5 days, or are boiled in milk. In traditional medicine strychnine is used for various purposes, as appetite stimulant, for the treatment of heartburns, insomnia, migraines or constipation. In constipation treatment strychnine activates peristalsis by acting on a neuro-muscular junction in bowel. By affecting vagus nerve strychnine increases hart rate, and sharpens all senses, for what it is considered as a general stimulant. As such, strychnine was often used for doping in sports and in very small concentrations it is added to some energy drinks. Strychnine is effective in treating impotency and improvement of the sexual desire.

Modern medical application of strychnine implies its use in heart failure, when massive doses are administrated. It is further used in the treatment of tetanus and cholera and has a promising potential for the treatment of functional forms of paralysis, facial neuralgia, epilepsy and atony. In toxicology strychnine is sometimes used as an antidote in poisoning with morphine and opium.

4. TROPANE ALKALOIDS

Tropane alkaloids are found in more than 3000 plant species of Solanaceae family. *Datura* plants pose a health risk primarily to livestock because they can contaminate feed crops, particularly soybean and linseed. The highest concentration of tropane alkaloids is found in roots and seeds of *Datura* species and the content of alkaloids vary depending on the plant age, location and weather conditions.

Medicinally most important tropane alkaloids are scopolamine, hyoscyamine and atropine, which represents a racemic mixture of l- and d-hyoscyamine.

Symptoms of poisoning with tropane alkaloids manifest 30 – 60 minutes upon ingestion and can last up to 48 hours. Intoxicated individuals are photophobic, confused and agitated and have dry mouth (Bliss, 2001). Urination is difficult to perform and after recovery individuals hardly recall the events due to amnesia.

Tropane alkaloids are important antidotes in cholinergic poisoning caused by organophosphorous pesticides and sarin, inhibiting neural signals transmitted by acetylcholine. *Scopolamine* is used as antiemetic to prevent nausea and vomiting associated with travel sickness and chemotherapy. Alkaloid is also used in ophthalmology for diagnostic procedures and in preoperative and postoperative states. *Hyoscyamine* in sulphate form is used clinically to treat a variety of stomach/intestinal problems such as cramps, bladder and bowel control problems. *Atropine* in the form of its sulfate salt may also be used for spastic conditions of the gastrointestinal tract, but the preference is given to hyoscyamine due to extreme toxicity of atropine.

Cocaine is another tropane alkaloid produced in *Erythroxylum coca* and *Erythroxylum truxillense*. Coca leaves, chewed or masticated with lime to improve buccal absorption, are used in some parts of Latin America as an energizer. The alkaloid has paralyzing effect on sensory nerve endings but is too toxic to be used as parenteral anesthetic. For this reason cocaine and numerous semisynthetic derivatives, like benzocaine, procaine, are only used as local anesthetics. Cocaine hydrochloride is used as local anesthetic in ophthalmology, face, nose, and throat surgery.

5. SOLANUM ALKALOIDS

Solanum alkaloids are produced by plants from Solanaceae family (*Atropa belladonna, Datura*, chili pepper, potato, tomato, eggplant, e.g.). *Datura* and belladona predominantly produce tropane alkaloids like atropine, hyoscyamine, cocaine and scopolamine, but are also able to produce other chemical groups of alkaloids. Solanum alkaloids are present in all parts of the plants, including leaves, roots, flowers, stems, and fruits, being a part of plant defense mechanism against insects and predators. The highest contents are observed in unripe fruit. Solanine (Figure IV.4) is known for its pesticidal properties and solanine-based insecticides have been produced, however the procedure for its isolation is quite expensive to be applied on industrial scale.

Most of solanum alkaloids occur as steroidal glycosides. The glycoalkaloids appear to be synthesized in the above-ground parts of the plants, not in the roots as is the case of tropane alkaloids.

Solanum alkaloids exhibit their toxicity via different mechanisms. Tomatine complexes membrane sterols causing pore formation and leakage of cell content, whereas solanine affects potassium channels in mitochondria initiating calcium transport from mitochondria to cytoplasm (Driniaev et al., 1980). Increased concentration of calcium in cytoplasm triggers cell damage and apoptosis. Several solanum alkaloids demonstrate antifungal effects, however some fungi have developed enzymes, like tomatinase, to inactivate alkaloids.

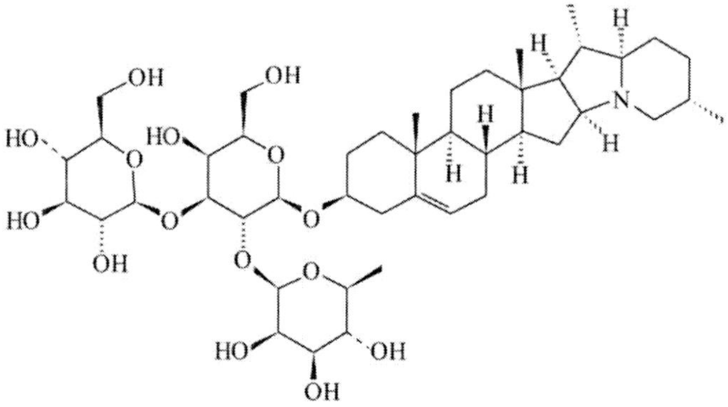

Figure IV.4. Solanine.

Solanine content is high in unripe potatoes and its production is also favored when the plant is damaged or exposed to a light, reaching the contents above 1 mg/g. A bitter taste and green color of potatoes, which originates from chlorophyll and plants biochemical battle, can indicate the processes undergoing in the plant and can alert elevated solanine content. Solanine is quite thermally stable so reduction of solanine content after frying can be attributed to extraction by fats. Other culinary processes, such as boiling or microwave heating, do not influence the content significantly.

Solanine demonstrates low oral acute toxicity due to poor absorption in gastrointestinal tract (Dalvi and Bowie, 1983). The compound is removed from the body fairly rapidly preventing its accumulation in tissues. Intestinal bacteria aid in detoxification by hydrolyzing the glycoside into its aglycone solanidine, which is less toxic than solanine.

The main target systems of solanine toxicity are gastrointestinal, cardiovascular and bones. The symptoms of solanine poisoning start demonstrating 6-8 hours upon ingestion, but the cases of symptoms development after, as quickly as 30 minutes, have been reported (Cantwell, 1996). In animal studies acute poisoning with solanine was accompanied with agitation, paralysis and hallucination, which were caused by acetylcholine build-up in synapses due to inhibited cholinesterase (Patil et al., 1972). Individuals intoxicated with solanine reported fever, throat burning, skin warming and flushing, dizziness and drowsiness. In prolonged studies solanine indicated teratogenicity provoking birth defects, like spina bifida (Mun et al., 1975).

In chronic exposure solanine acts as endocrine disruptor especially to thyroid, and contributes to joint inflammation, arthritis development and osteoporosis (Patil et al., 1972). Solanine effects on bones can be explained by its ability to remove calcium from bones and deposit it in any predisposed area in the body. Removed calcium can also be deposited in blood vessels contributing to arteriosclerosis.

There is no antidote available for solanine poisoning. To reduce its absorption from gastrointestinal tract gastric lavage and administration of activated charcoal are useful. To control convulsions diazepams are administrated.

In folk medicine due to sedative and anticonvulsant properties solanine was used in the treatment of epilepsy and asthma, as well as for cough relieve. Chaconine has shown nematocidal effects, whereas solamargine demonstrated potent cytotoxicity to cancerous human hepatocytes and skin fibroblasts (Andersson, 1999).

REFERENCES

Andersson, C. Glycoalkaloids in *Tomatoes, Eggplants, Pepper and Two Solanum Species growing wild in the Nordic countries*. Nordic Council of Ministers, Copenhagen, 1999.

Bliss, M. Datura Plant Poisoning. *Clin Tox Rev* 23 (6), 2001.

Driniaev VA, Troshko EV, Artiushkova VA, Kulida LI. Nature and mechanism of action of the solanidine glycosides solanine and chaconine on biological objects. *Nauchnye Doki Vyss Shkoly Biol Nauki*. 10, 1980,5-16.

Cantwell M. A Review of Important Facts about Potato Glycoalkaloids. *Perish Hand News* 87, 1996, 26-27.

Chapman RA and Miller DJ. The effects of caffeine on the contraction of the frog heart. *J Physiol*. 242(3), 1974, 589–613.

Dalvi RR and Bowie WC. Toxicology of solanine: an overview. *Vet Hum Tox*. 25(1), 1983, 13-15.

De Costa C. St Anthony's Fire and living ligatures: a short history of ergometrine. *The Lancet* 359, 2002.1768-1770.

Eadie MJ. Convulsive ergotism: epidemics of the serotonin syndrome? *The Lancet Neurology* 2 (7), 2003, 429-434.

Emerman CL, Devlin C, Connors AF. Risk of toxicity in patients with elevated theophylline levels. *Ann Emerg Med.* 19(6), 1990, 643-648.

Gallo RV, Rabii J, Moberg GP. Effect of methysergide, a blocker of serotonin receptors, on plasma prolactin levels in lactating and ovariectomized rats. *Endocrinology* 97(5), 1975, 1096-1105.

Gupta, RC, *Handbook of Toxicology of Chemical Warfare Agents,* Elsevier Inc., 2009.

Halpern JH and Harrison GP. Hallucinogen persisting perception disorder: what do we know after 50 years? *Drug Alcohol Dep* 69 (2), 2003, 109-119.

Miyakawa N, Uchino S, Yamashita T, Okada H, Nakamura T, Kaminogawa S, Miyamoto Y, Hisatsune T. A glycine receptor antagonist, strychnine, blocked NMDA receptor activation in the neonatal mouse neocortex. *Neuroreport.* 13(13), 2002, 1667-1673.

Mun AM, Barden ES, Wilson JM, Hogan JM. Teratogenic effects in early chick embryos of solanine and glycoalkaloids from potatoes infected with late-blight, Phytophthora infestans. *Teratology.* 11(1), 1975, 73-78.

Patil BC, Sharma RP, Salunkhe DK, Salunkhe K. Evaluation of solanine toxicity. *Food Cosm Tox.* 10(3), 1972, 395-398.

Rowell PP and Larson BT. Ergocryptine and other ergot alkaloids stimulate the release of [3H] dopamine from rat striatal synaptosomes. *J Anim Sci* 77(7), 1999, 1800-1806.

Samuelsson, G. *Drugs of natural origin.* 4th ed. Apotekar societeten, 1999, Stockholm.

Sanders SW, Haering H.Mosberg H, Jaeger H. Pharmacokinetics of ergotamine in healthy volunteers following oral and rectal dosing. *Eur J Clin Pharm* 30(3), 1986, 331-334.

Sharma RK. *Consice textbook of forensic medicine & toxicology*, Elsevier, 2008.

Chapter V

ADVERSE EFFECTS OF NATURAL PHENOLS

More than 4000 natural phenolic compounds have been identified differing in their structure significantly and encompassing from simple to highly condensed molecules. For natural phenolic compounds mostly beneficial effects are promoted and claimed, however under certain circumstances some compounds may pose a health risk to humans and livestock. Health promoting effects attributed to natural phenols include anti-viral, anti-allergic, anti-inflammatory, anti-proliferative, anti-carcinogenic and other effects (Bravo, 1998; Wojdyło et al., 2007; Yoon and Baek, 2006; Stoner and Mukhtar, 1995). Antioxidant effects of natural phenols arise from their ability to scavenge free radicals by becoming radicals themselves through formation of resonantly stabilized radical species (Figure V.1).

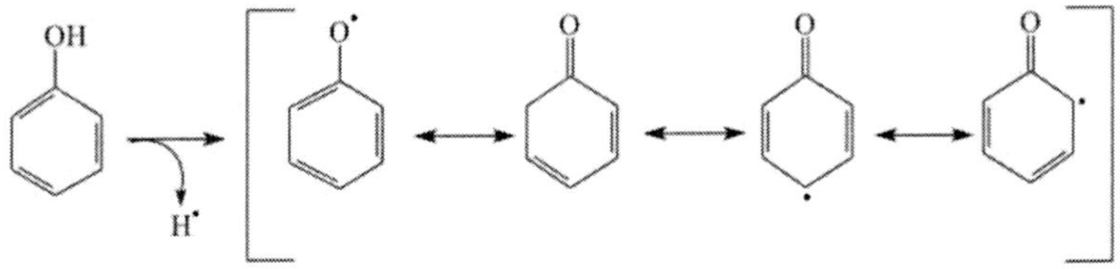

Figure V.1. Resonance stabilization of phenols.

By scavenging reactive radicals that are formed in the body, phenols prevent cell damage and cell proliferation, which are often in the core of carcinogenesis, as well as the disturbance of lipid metabolism responsible for cardiovascular diseases. Dietary phenols inhibit formation of carcinogenic nitrosamines from ingested nitrites and nitrates. Following similar mechanism as scavenging of free radicals, natural phenols can trap reactive electrophiles. Electrophiles can also damage the cells by reacting with essential molecules. Another effect attributed to phenols is inhibition of prostaglandin formation. Prostaglandins are important endogenous molecules produced from arachidonic acid that regulate the contraction and relaxation of smooth muscle tissue and act locally as messenger molecules.

Even diverse in their structure, all phenols are structurally related, they contain one or more benzene rings with one or more hydroxyl group substitutions. Their major classes include:

- Phenolic acids:
  Hydroxybenzoic acids
  Hydroxycinnamic acids
- Flavonoids:
  Antocyanins
  Proantocyanidins
  Flavonols
  Flavones
  Flavanols
  Flavanones
  Isoflavones
- Stilbenes
- Lignans

1. MAJOR CLASSES OF NATURAL PHENOLS

Phenolic acids are either derivatives of benzoic or cinnamic acid. The content of hydroxybenzoic acids in edible plants is generally low, with the exception of onion, red fruits and black radish. In general, derivatives of benzoic acid are found in few plants and for this are not extensively studied. Gallotannins are oligomers of gallic acid and are high in mangoes. Ellagitannins are abundantly presents in strawberries, raspberries and blackberries.

Derivatives of cinnamic acid (Figure V.2) are more common than hydroxybenzoic acid derivatives. In food they are rarely found in their free form, only in processed food (freezing, fermentation, sterilization). p-Coumaric acid lowers the risk of stomach cancer by reducing the formation of nitrosamines. Chlorogenic acid is produced from its precursor, a caffeic acid, and is high in instant coffee. The compound has the effect to release glucose into the blood after a meal. Ferulic acid is abundant in outer parts of the grains, so its content in flour is related to sieving. Rice and oat contain approximate contents of ferulic acid, whereas in maize its content is three fold higher.

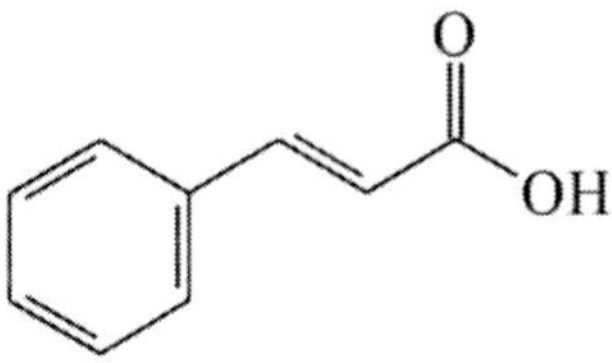

Figure V.2. Cinnamic acid.

Flavonoids have a common structure composed of two aromatic rings bound with oxygenated heterocycle (Figure V.3). The compounds are abundant in citrus plants. More than 60 flavonoids have been identified and they have been divided into 14 classes. Most abundant classes of flavonoids include:

- Flavonols
- Flavanones
- Isoflavones
- Flavanols
- Lignans
- Stilbenes

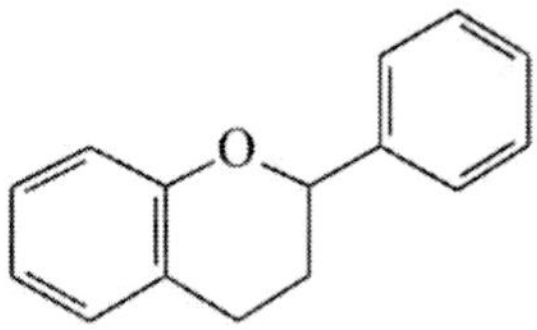

Figure V.3. Common skeleton of flavonoids.

Flavonols accumulate in outer tissues of plants, such as skin and leaves, because their synthesis is stimulated by light. In leafy vegetables like cabbage their concentration in outer leaves may be up to ten times greater. It is not uncommon for their concentration to differ at different sides of the same fruit.

The main sources of *flavanones* are citrus fruits, where polymethoxylated compounds, such as sinessetin, haxamethoxyflavone, nobiletin, scutellarein, heptamethoxyflavone and tangererin, are found. Main aglycones are naringenin, hesperetin and eridictyol. Albedo and membranes of citrus fruits have the highest quantity of flavanones. For this reason fruit juice may contain up to five times less phenols than the whole fruit. Glycosides with neohesperidose, like those in grapefruit, have bitter taste, while those with rutinose are mostly flavorless.

Isoflavones have phenyl ring attached in position 3 rather than in position 2 (Figure V.4). This class of flavonoids is most investigated for demonstrating pseudo hormonal properties due to structural similarities with estrogens. Soybean and other leguminous plants represent the richest sources of isoflavonoids. Most important phytoestrogens are genistein, daidzein, glycitein, biochanin A and formononetin.

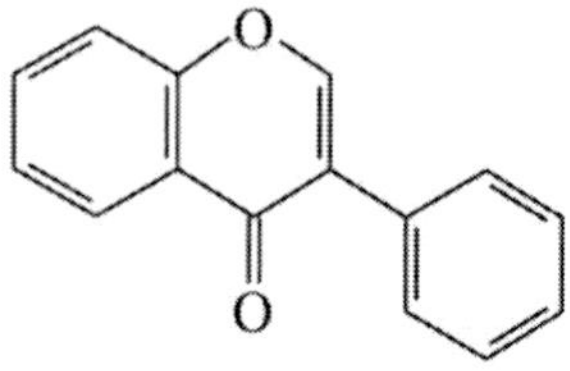

Figure V.4. Common skeleton of isoflavones.

Flavanols are not normally glycosylated. Catechins are their monomeric forms, whereas proanthocyanidins represent polymeric form.

Lignans in their glycoside form are about thousand times higher in flaxseed than in other plants. The compounds are composed of two phenylpropanoid units (C6-C3) and act like phytoestrogens. Lignans have anti-estrogenic properties and can reduce the risk of hormone-related cancers. When part of human diet, some lignans are metabolized by the activity of intestinal bacteria to form mammalian lignans known as enterodiol and enterolactone.

Stilbene derivatives, especially *trans* isomers, have also estrogenic activity and are used in the production of non-steroidal synthetic estrogens. This class of flavonoids is high in Pinaceae, Myrtaceae and Moraceae generas.

In plants heartwood normally stilbene aglycones are present, whereas in other plant tissues stilbenes are in the form of glycosides.

2. GOSSYPOL

Gossypol is a yellow, toxic compound found in stems, seed and root of a cotton plant, where it serves to fight pests. Among *Gossypium* L. species *Gossypium hirsutum* is mostly grown for fiber production. Cotton seed is rich in proteins and oil and is used for oil and feed production. After fiber removal cottonseed is crushed or extracted. China and India are major producers of cotton, but the crop is also intensively produced in Pakistan and Brazil. In Europe the largest producers are Turkey and Greece. The seeds of Gossipium species vary in gossypol content remarkably with gossypol being in the range 0.13- 10%. Many attempts have been made to reduce gossypol content in the cotton seed. In transgenic cotton genes coding *Bacillus thuringiensis* insecticidal proteins have been introduced. Glandless cotton lacks in glands that produce gossypol, however this variety is commercially inviable because it is very prone to pests.

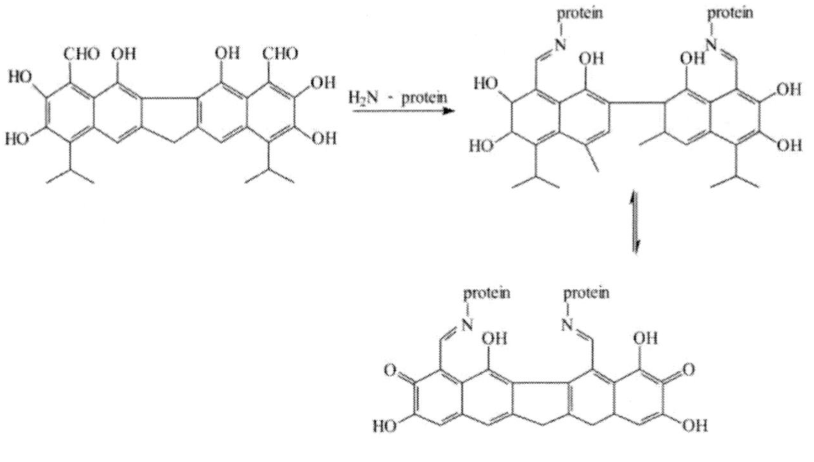

Figure V.5. Gossypol interaction with proteins.

Gossypol exhibits chirality because the molecule is non-planar. Levorotary enantiomer is more biologically active, however dextrorotary is more slowly eliminated from the body prolonging its effects. The compound readily reacts with amines and amino groups of proteins, forming the bound form which is less toxic (Figure V.5). The reaction is accelerated by heat and moisture, but the bound gossypol is also formed spontaneously during the storage of the cottonseed. Bound form complexes some metals reducing their bioavailability in feed.

In some Asian countries like China cotton is a primary source of edible oil. First observations related to toxicity of the cotton oil were made in 40` in China when extremely low birth rates were reported. Farmers that consumed homemade unheated cotton oil developed fatigue and burning sensation on the face. The effects were attributed to gossypol. Later on it was established that gossypol inhibits enzymes that play a crucial role in energy generation in sperm and spermatogenic cells (Shaaban et al., 2008). For its effects on reproduction, gossypol gained popularity as a principal contraceptive method in China in 70`. Gossypol was effective also in female animals, in which abortifacient effects resulting from consumption of feed based on the cotton seed cake were documented.

Gossypol affects metabolism of other compounds by binding to microsomal membranes decreasing the activity of cytochrome P450 and cytochrome b5 enzymes, NADPH- cytochrome c-reductase and aminopyrine N-demethylase, as well as aniline hydroxylase (Abou-Donia, 1976). The metabolism is affected also by depletion of iron and glutathione. Pro-oxidant effects of gossypol are caused by oxidative stress.

Symptoms of acute poisoning with gossypol include difficulty in breathing due to pulmonary edema. The fluid is accumulated not only in thoracic but also in peritoneal cavity. Death occurs due to circulatory failure because gossypol prevents oxygen release from oxyhemoglobin (Abou-Donia, 1976).

In large scale study conducted in China and involving 8000 males gossypol was tested as antifertility agent in doses 20 mg of racemic mixture per day (Liu, 1985). The compound was efficient and well tolerated, did not cause changes in major biochemical parameters and blood pressure, but caused hypokalemia in 10% of tested individuals. Second conducted study included 151 man and lower doses. 15 mg of (±) gossypol was administrated daily for 12-16 weeks and during next 40 weeks the dose was reduced to 10 mg of (±) gossypol/day. Spermatogenesis suppression was observed in 53% of the tested individuals (Coutinho, 2002). After 12 month upon study cessation 51% of individuals recovered sperm count, whereas 18% remained azoospermic.

Human trials were also conducted in females, because it was noticed that women consuming homemade cottonseed oil suffered from burning fever and atrophy of the uterus. Women participating in the trial suffered from endometriosis, uterine myomas or uterine bleeding. 20 mg of (±) gossypol was administrated daily for 2-3 month and next 4-5 month the dose was increased to 40 mg of (±) gossypol/day. As a result an atrophy of endometrium and other cytotoxic effects in uterus, as well as systematic effects on ovarian function, were observed (Zhu, 1984).

In *in vitro* studies gossypol demonstrated some beneficial effects. In cell lines of breast, colon, prostate cancer and leukemia, gossypol inhibited cell growth. Proposed mechanism included inhibition of enzymes involved in DNA replication and repair of cancerous cells. It was shown that gossypol uncouples oxidative phosphorilation that occurs at mitochondrial membranes and is important for the production of adenosine triphosphate (ATP) (Balakrishnan et al., 2008). Currently phase I and II clinical trials are being conducted in respect to gossypol influence on Non-Hodgkin lymphoma, breast and prostate cancer. In addition, gossypol-based topical spermicides are available and the compound may be used as a part of a therapy for transsexual patients.

Due to recognized effects on reproduction it is important to consider gossypol content in feed. During oil removal from the cotton seed, either mechanically or by extraction, free gossypol is mostly eliminated. Further exposure to heat reduces gossypol content for 9-12%, whereas exposure for ten minutes to steam results in 62% gossypol reduction (Barraza et al., 1991; Danke and Tilman, 1965). Extrusion, in addition to gossypol reduction, alters protein digestibility and lysine bioavailability. Free gossypol can further be reduced in feed by addition of iron salts which complexes free gossypol. Ingested via feed gossypol can further be transferred to edible animal parts indirectly exposing consumers. Transfer rates of free gossypol from feed to animal parts used in human diet are unknown, nor the bioavailability of gossypol bound in edible tissues. Expected concentrations are expected to be of negligible risk to consumers.

3. PHLORIZIN

Phlorizin (Figure V.6) was first isolated from the bark of the apple tree in 1835 by French chemist. The compound belongs to the chalcone class and has a bitter taste, for what its antipyretic and anti-malaria properties were assumed.

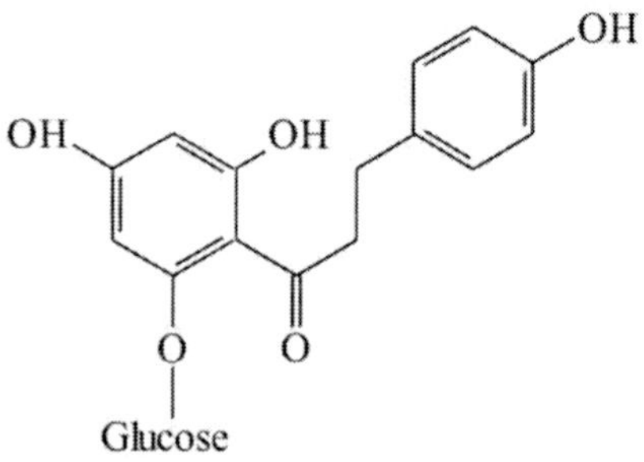

Figure V.6. Phlorizin.

In apples phlorizin makes about 11-36% of total phenolics, but the compound is also found in other fruits, like cherry and pear. In plants phlorizin serves to regulate the growth and development. Its dimerized oxidation products are responsible for a color of the apple fruit. Phloretin is an aglycone of phlorizin which acts as fungicide in plants, and in humans it produces relaxation of coronary artery rings.

Phlorizin is being used in medical practice for more than 150 years due to its potent effects to resemble glycosuria. There are several types of glycosuria. In pregnancy slightly elevated renal glucose is normally to be expected. Elevated glucose concentrations in urine can occur in normal carbohydrate metabolism in the absence of hyperglycemia or can be dependent on the amount of ingested carbohydrates. Phlorizin causes glycosuria without affecting blood glucose.

The mechanism by which phlorizin affects glucose levels is via affecting glucose transporters, mostly in renal tubules (White and Pharm, 2010). Phlorizin affinity to glucose transporters is 1000 – 3000 times greater of that for glucose. Specialized glucose transporters carry glucose against concentration gradient by coupling glucose transport with sodium transport. Several forms of sodium-linked glucose transporters (SGLT) exist. Type 1 (SGLT 1) transporters couple two molecules of glucose with one sodium ion, whereas those of type 2 (SGLT-2) symport one glucose with one sodium.

SGLT-1 transporters are located primarily in small intestine wall and distal segments of renal tubular epithelium. These transporters have low capacity to glucose, but high affinity. Phlorizin has affinity to sodium-linked glucose transporters of type 1 about two orders of magnitude greater in comparison to SGLT-2. Type 2 transporters are low affinity glucose-sodium cotransporters located in proximal convoluted renal tubule. SGLT 1 transporters are able to transports both glucose and galactose, whereas SGLT-2 transport only glucose. Phlorizin influences glucose levels without affecting sodium gradient. The compound also influences glucose uptake by brain. The mechanism of such effect is still unclear because blood-brain barrier does not employ sodium-glucose symporters.

Other effects of phlorizin have also been recognized. The transport of toxic cycasin is inhibited in the presence of phlorizin (Matsuoka et al., 1998). Cycasin is a toxic principle from the seeds of several species of *Cycas* palms, native to Guam. The compound acts like neurotoxin and is neoplastic to liver, kidneys, intestines, and lungs. In memory impairment phlorizin antagonizes insulin (Boccia et al., 1999). After administrating phlorizin into proximal convoluted tubule it was noticed that phlorizin affects reabsorption of sodium, potassium, chloride and water in distal convoluted tubules.

Upon ingestion phlorizin is very rapidly converted to phloretin with 90% conversion by hydrolysis catalyzed by lactose-phlorizin hydrolase, located in small intestine epithelial cells (Ehrenkranz et al., 2005). The enzyme catalyzes lactose hydrolysis as well. Lactose-intolerant individuals are expected to have decreased phlorizin conversion. Phloretin itself is bioactive exhibiting estrogenic activity and influencing the bioavailability of other substances. The compound inhibits facilitative transporters of glucose, galactose and fructose in the gut, uncouples mitochondrial oxidative phosphorilation and inhibits membrane transport of chloride, bicarbonate and lithium in erythrocytes.

For its effects on lowering blood glucose independently on insulin, phlorizin is nowadays considered as attractive natural agent for the treatment of type 2 diabetes because it reduces blood glucose without the risk of hypoglycemia. Phlorizin is attractive for treating obesity because it blocs glucose reabsorption reducing caloric intake. The compound is used for diagnostic purposes in non-invasive clearance method for measuring glomerular filtration rate and renal blood flow rate. The method was developed in 1930 by Homer Smith (Smith, 1943).

4. RESVERATROL

Resveratrol (Figure V.7) is stilbenoid first isolated from *Veratrum album*, a medicinal plant of the Liliaceae family native to Europe. The compound exists in *cis* and *trans* form and in plants is often bound to glucose. Animal studies conducted up to date and oriented to revealing resveratrol effects, were primarily focused on elucidating its anti-cancer and anti-inflammatory effects. Blood sugar lowering properties were speculated and several human trials, involving high doses of resveratrol have been conducted. In one of such trials 250 mg/day of resveratrol was administrated to patients with type 2 diabetes what showed to be effective in improving glycemic control (Bhatt et al., 2012).

In plants resveratrol is synthetized with the aid of resveratrol-synthase. The compound is high in red grapes, cocoa, peanuts and blueberries. Upon ingestion up to 70% of resveratrol is absorbed, however its bioavailability is very low because the compound is rapidly metabolized in intestines and liver to glucuronate and sulfate metabolites, among which mainly represented are *trans*-resveratrol-3-O-glucuronide and *trans*-resveratrol-3-sulfate (Yu et al., 2002; la Porte et al., 2010).

In conducted studies resveratrol extended the lifespan of yeast (*Saccharomices cerevisiae*), worms (*Caenorhabditis elegans*) and fruit fly (*Drosophila melanogaster*) (Wood et al., 2004). In vertebrates the lifespan and activity of short-lived fish (*Nothobranchius furzeri*) was increased by 56% (Valenzano et al., 2006).Fish had higher swimming activity and better learning, however slight increase in mortality in young fish was observed. In mice resveratrol reduced mortality caused by high fat diet for 30%, but did not influence blood cholesterol and triglycerides. In *in vitro* studies resveratrol inhibited replication of type 1 and 2 herpes simplex virus (HSV), influenza viruses, human cytomegalovirus, respiratory viruses and varicellar virus (Docherty et al., 1999).

Special focus was put on potential anticarcinogenic effects of resveratrol. In mice treated with carcinogentopical application of resveratrol prevented skin cancer development (Athar et al., 2007). In rats 1 mg/kg of orally administrated resveratrol reduced the number and size of esophageal tumors (Li et al., 2002). Pterostilbene (Figure V.7), a dimethylether derivative of resveratrol, has gained increasing attention as a potential cancer chemopreventive agent against colon cancer due to longer half-life in comparison to resveratrol. In conducted *in vivo* experiments 0.02-8 mg/kg of orally administrated pterostilbene prevented the development of intestinal and colon tumors, inhibiting colon cancer cell growth and colony formation (Nutakul et al., 2011). The compound was ineffective in other tumor types.

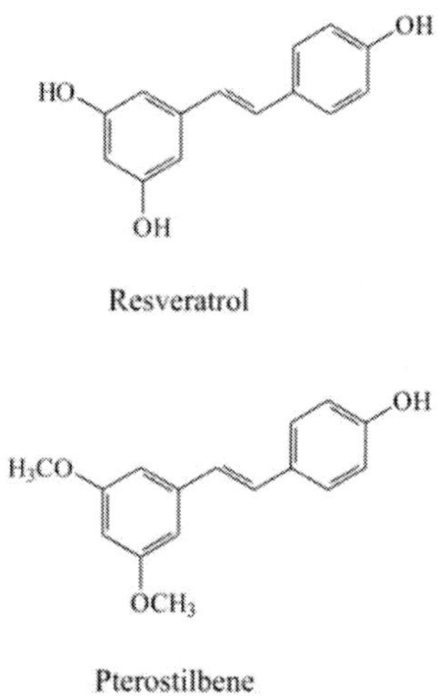

Resveratrol

Pterostilbene

Figure V.7. Resveratrol and its derivative.

Resveratrol interferes with all three stages of carcinogenesis – initiation, promotion and progression. Several mechanisms have been proposed for resveratrol influence on cancer formation and development. It is postulated that resveratrol enhances nuclear transcription factor kappa (NF-kB) which suppresses carcinogenesis because kappa light chains are key components of immunoglobulin's involved in cell response to free radicals, UV, bacteria's and viruses (Leiro et al., 2005). Incorrect regulation of the nuclear transcription factor kappa has been linked to cancer and autoimmune diseases. Other studies suggest that resveratrol inhibits the progression of breast cancer by the same mechanisms as anticancer drugs, namely by affecting topoisomerase that regulates overwinding and underwinding of DNA (Leone et al., 2010). Taking into consideration proposed mechanism it is recommended to take precaution with resveratrol in pregnancy. Furthermore, it was observed that resveratrol supplements can interfere with oral contraceptives.

Beneficial effects of resveratrol in cardio protection are explained by different mechanisms. It is believed that resveratrol inhibits the expression of vascular cell adhesion molecules and vascular smooth muscle cell proliferation. Furthermore, resveratrol stimulates endothelial nitric oxide synthase activity, inhibits lipid peroxidation and platelet aggregation (Li et al., 2002). Nitric oxide synthase catalyzes the production of nitric oxide from L-arginine, requiring several cofactors – NADPH, FAD, FMN and heme. Nitric oxide is important cell signaling molecule that conducts intracellular signals that control vascular tone, insulin secretion, peristalsis and angiogenesis.

It is believed that resveratrol supplements can be beneficial in patients with Alzheimer's disease, because in animal studies oral administration of resveratrol reduced beta amyloid plaque formation in brain, probably chelating copper (Karuppagounder et al., 2009). Resveratrol dietary supplements are available in the range of resveratrol contents, form 50% to 99%. Due to poor oral bioavailability supplements are also available in chewing gum formulation for buccal absorption. In addition to discussed effects supplements are promoted for analgetic purposes, because resveratrol inhibits cyclooxygenase. Common analgesics, like aspirin and ibuprofen, work according to same principle. Cyclooxygenase is responsible for the formation of inflammatory mediators, like prostaglandins, prostacyclins and tromboxane from arachidonic acid. Long-term effects of taking resveratrol supplements are unknown. Acute overdoses may cause stomach cramping, reduced appetite, excitation, tingling and numbness. The effects subside few days after taking resveratrol.

5. HYDROXYTYROSOL

Hydroxytyrosol (Figure V.8) is colorless, odorless liquid compound found in olive leaves and other plant parts. In olive oil hydoxytyrosol, together with oleuropein, contributes to built-up of bitterness. The content of hydoxytyrosol in olives depends on the cultivar, soil, climate and degree of olives ripeness. Hydroxytyrosol is considered to be one of the most powerful antioxidants, having antioxidant potential twice of that of quercetin and three times of epicatechin.

Most frequently cited beneficial health effects linked to hydoxytyrosol include reduced oxidative stress, anticancer effects, prevention of lipid peroxidation and neuroprotective effects (González-Correa et al., 2008). In *in vitro* experiments hydoxytyrosol inhibited proliferation of leukemia and human colon cancer cell lines and induced apoptosis (Fabiani et al., 2006). The effects were not observed in normal cells. Neuroprotective effect is believed to occur due to influence on mitochondria of the brain cells. To brain cells hydoxytyrosol is transported via passive diffusion and is degraded to homovanillic alcohol.

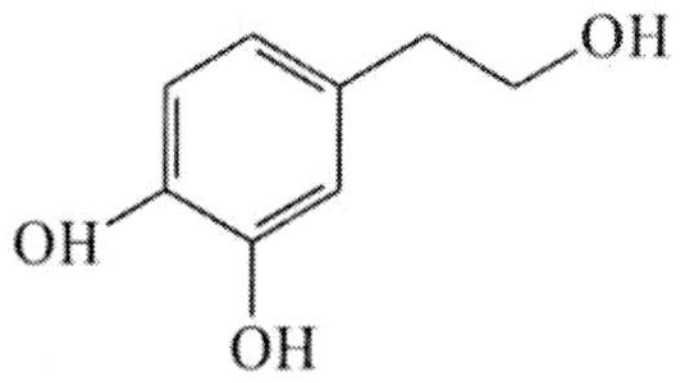

Figure V.8. Hydroxytyrosol.

After absorption hydoxytyrosol is rapidly biotransformed by catechol-O-methyltransferase, alcohol dehydrogenase, aldehyde dehydrogenase and phenolsulfotransferase of blood cells and other tissues. The compound is rapidly distributed mostly to lungs, kidneys and liver, and is able to cross blood/brain barrier. Uptake by brain is slower when compared to other organs (Angelo et al., 2001).

By FDA hydoxytyrosol is recognized as GRAS (Generally Recognized as Safe) and is used as food preservative, especially for fish products. Hydroxytyrosol is available in the form of dietary supplements for general health.

6. CAFFEIC AND FERULIC ACIDS

Caffeic acid is found in all plants and is a precursor to ferulic acid and synapyl alcohol (Figure V.9) being involved in lignin synthesis. As a pure compound it is used as black and white photographic developer and in MALDI MS (Matrix-Assisted Laser Desorption Ionization Mass spectrometry) analysis. Its phenethyl ester is one of the active compounds in propolis responsible for its anti-inflammatory effects. Anti-metastatic and anti-tumor effects were also attributed to this phenethyl ester. Both caffeic and chlorogenic acids reduce DNA methylation responsible for tumor growth (Lee and Zhu, 2004). The speculations of anticarcinogenic effects of caffeic acid are contradictory because some animal experiments demonstrated opposite effects. Oral administration of caffeic acid in rats produced stomach papillomas, what was explained by the formation of different metabolites by rat gut bacteria (Hirose et al., 1998). Caffeic acid exhibits anti-inflammatory effects by inhibiting lipoxygenase that is responsible for the formation of leukotriens from arachidonic acid (Mirzoeva et al., 1995).

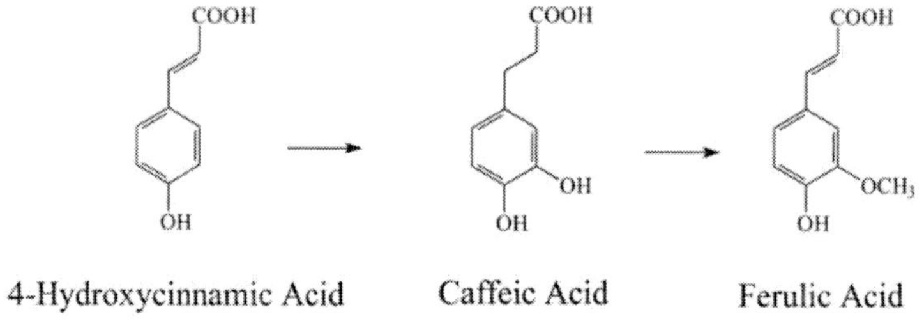

4-Hydroxycinnamic Acid   Caffeic Acid   Ferulic Acid

Figure V.9. Formation of ferulic acid via caffeic acid.

Ferulic acid is formed from caffeic acid by the activity of O-methyltransferase (Figure V.9). In plants ferulic acid serves to crosslink lignin with polysaccharides and to give rigidity to the cell walls. Acai fruit, from acai palm, which produces small black berries, is particularly rich natural source of ferulic acid. Industrially ferulic acid is used for the production of vanillin and in MALDI MS analysis.

Antitumor effect of ferulic acid was observed in animal studies and *in vitro*, particularly against liver, tongue, lung, colon, prostate and breast cancer. Ferulic acid demonstrated pro-apoptotic effects in cancer cells (Valentão et al., 2011). In other *in vitro* experiments the compound has demonstrated to inactivate superoxide, nitric oxide and hydroxyl radicals (Cano et al., 2002). Antioxidant effects of ferulic acid are particularly pronounced on skin and the compound is intensively used as a component of anti-aging skin care products and sunscreens. It is believed that ferulic acid reduces menopausal symptoms and protects against bone degeneration.

7. ANTRAQUINONES

Antraquinones are synthetized by many plants of *Fabeaceae, Liliaceae, Rhamnaceae* and *Polygonacea* families, like senna, rhubarb, yellow dock, aloe vera, frangula and others. The plants are used as cathartics, laxatives and purgatives. Cathartics and purgatives accelerate defecation in contrast to laxatives, which ease defecation. Cathartic effect may be produced by other natural compounds as well, such as saponins, tannins, volatile oils and alkaloids.

Antraquinones are phenolic compounds of C6-C2-C6 structure, often yellow and bitter. In many plants during storage their dimmers and condensed forms are formed, which are less bioactive. For this reason antraquinones producing plants are prior use stored for prolonged period in order to reduce the potency and to avoid violent and painful defecation. On contrast to condensed forms dynamic isomers anthron and anthranol are more bioactive (Figure V.10).

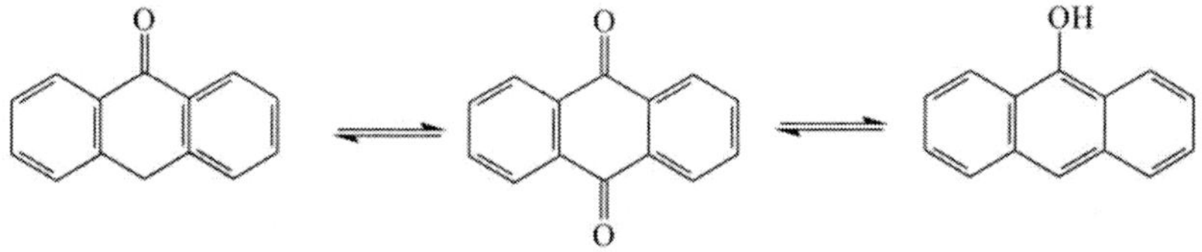

| Anthron | Antraquinone | Anthranol |

Figure V.10. Antraquinone and its dynamic isomers.

Antraquinones of Cascara Sagrada (*Rhamnus purshianus*) are known as cascarosides and are found in both *O*- and *C*-glycoside forms. In plant bark cascarosides make up 60%. The bark has long tradition of being used as cathartic. Once stripped from the tree, the bark is aged for about one year to make its effect milder. Effects of cascarosides are observed 8-10h after ingestion and are both local and systematic. Namely, gut flora hydrolyses glycosides producing prostaglandins, which effect nerve endings in the gut wall (Švarc-Gajić, 2011). In addition to their cathartic effects, cascarosides increase the bile flow easing the digestion. FDA has classified Cascara Sagrada preparations as genotoxic and/or carcinogenic, so their use is not recommended in pregnancy.

REFERENCES

Abou-Donia MB. Physiological effects and metabolism of gossypol. *Residue Rev.* 61, 1976, 125-160.

Angelo S, Manna C, Migliardi V, Mazzoni O, Capasso G, Pontoni G, Galletti G, Zappia V. Pharmacokinetics and Metabolism of Hydroxytyrosol, a

Natural Antioxidant from Olive Oil. *Drug Met Disp.* 29(11), 2001,1492-1498.

Athar M, Back JH, Tang X, Kim KH, Kopelovich L, Bickers DR, Kim AL. Resveratrol: a review of preclinical studies for human cancer prevention. *Tox Appl Pharm.* 224 (3), 2007, 274–283.

Balakrishnan K, Wierda WG, Keating MJ, Gandhi V. Gossypol, a BH3 mimetic, induces apoptosis in chronic lymphocytic leukemia cells. *Blood* 112, 2008, 1971-1980.

Barraza ML, Coppock CE, Brooks KN, Wilks DL, Saunders ED and Latimer WG. Iron sulphate and feed pelleting to detoxify free gossypol in cottonseed diet for dairy cattle. *J Dairy Sci* 74, 1991, 3457-3467.

Bhatt JK, Thomas S, Nanjan MJ. Resveratrol supplementation improves glycemic control in type 2 diabetes mellitus. *Nutr Res.* 32(7), 2012, 537-541.

Boccia MM, Kopf SR, Baratti CM. Phlorizin, a Competitive Inhibitor of Glucose Transport, Facilitates Memory Storage in Mice. *Neur Learn Mem.* 71(1), 1999, 104-112.

Bravo, L. Polyphenols: chemistry, dietary sources, metabolism, and nutritional significance. *Nutr Rev,* 56, 1998, 317-333.

Cano A, Arnao MB, Williamson G, Garcia-Conesa MT. Superoxide scavenging by polyphenols: effect of conjugation and dimerization. *Redox Rep.* 7(6), 2002, 379-83.

Coutinho EM. Gossypol: a contraceptive for men. *Contraception* 65, 2002, 259-263.

Danke RJ and Tilman D. Effect of free gossypol and supplemental dietary iron on blood constituents of rats. *J Nutr* 87, 1965, 493-498.

Docherty JJ, Fu MM, Stiffler BS, Limperos RJ, Pokabla CM, DeLucia AL. Resveratrol inhibition of herpes simplex virus replication. *Antiviral Res.* 43 (3), 1999, 145–155.

Ehrenkranz JRL, Lewis NG, Kahn CR. Phlorizin: a review. *Diabetes Met Res Rev* 21, 2005, 31–38.

Fabiani R, De Bartolomeo A, Rosignoli P, Servili M, Selvaggini R, Montedoro GF, Di Saverio C, Morozzi G. Virgin olive oil phenols inhibit proliferation of human promyelocytic leukemia cells (HL60) by inducing apoptosis and differentiation. *J Nutr.* 136(3), 2006, 614-619.

González-Correa JA, Navas MD, Lopez-Villodres JA, Trujillo M, Espartero JL, De La Cruz JP. Neuroprotective effect of hydroxytyrosol and hydroxytyrosol acetate in rat brain slices subjected to hypoxia-reoxygenation. *Neurosci Lett.* 446(2-3), 2008, 143-146.

Hirose M, Takesada Y, Tanaka H, Tamano S, Kato T, Shirai T. Carcinogenicity of antioxidants BHA, caffeic acid, sesamol, 4-methoxyphenol and catechol at low doses, either alone or in combination, and modulation of their effects in a rat medium-term multi-organ carcinogenesis model. *Carcinogenesis* 19 (1), 1998, 207–212.

Jo C, Yook HS, Lee MS, Kim JH, Song HP, Kwon JS, Byun MW, 2003. Irradiation effects on embryotoxicity and oxidative properties of gossypol dissolved in methanol. *Food Chem Tox.* 41, 1329-1336.

Karuppagounder SS, Pinto JT, Xu H, Chen HL, Beal MF, Gibson GE. Dietary supplementation with resveratrol reduces plaque pathology in a transgenic model of Alzheimer's disease. *Neurochem Int.* 54 (2), 2009, 111–118.

la Porte C, Voduc N, Zhang G, Seguin I, Tardiff D, Singhal N, Cameron DW. Steady-State pharmacokinetics and tolerability of trans-resveratrol 2000 mg twice daily with food, quercetin and alcohol (ethanol) in healthy human subjects. *Clin Pharmacokin* 49 (7), 2010, 449–454.

Lee WJ and Zhu BT.Strong inhibition of DNA methylation by caffeic acid and chlorogenic acid, two polyphenolic components present in coffee. *Proc Amer Assoc Cancer Res*, 45, 2004, 36-41.

Leiro J, Arranz JA, Fraiz N, Sanmartín ML, Quezada E, Orallo F. Effect of cis-resveratrol on genes involved in nuclear factor kappa B signaling. *Int Immunopharm* 5 (2), 2005, 393–406.

Leone S, Cornetta T, Basso E, Cozzi R. Resveratrol induces DNA double-strand breaks through human topoisomerase II interaction. *Cancer Lett.* 295(2), 2010, 167-172

Li ZG, Hong T, Shimada Y, Komoto I, Kawabe A, Ding Y, Kaganoi J, Hashimoto Y, Imamura M. Suppression of N-nitrosomethylbenzylamine (NMBA)-induced esophageal tumorigenesis in F344 rats by resveratrol. *Carcinogenesis* 23 (9), 2002, 1531–1536

Liu GZ. Clinical trial of gossypol as a male contraceptive: a randomized controlled study. *Zhonghua Yi Xue ZA Zhi* 65, 1985, 107-109.

Matsuoka T, Nishizaki T, Kisby GE. Na+-dependent and phlorizin-inhibitable transport of glucose and cycasin in brain endothelial cells. *J Neurochem.* 70(2), 1998, 772-727.

Mirzoeva OK, Sudina GF, Pushkareva MA, Korshunova GA, Sumbatian NV, Varfolomeev SD. Lipophilic derivatives of caffeic acid as lipoxygenase inhibitors with antioxidant properties. *Bioorg Khim.* 21(2), 1995,143-151.

Nutakul W, Sobers HS, Qiu P, Dong P, Decker EA, McClements DJ, Xiao H. Inhibitory Effects of Resveratrol and Pterostilbene on Human Colon

Cancer Cells: A Side-by-Side Comparison. *J Agric Food Chem.* 2011, 59, 10964–10970.

Shaaban WF, Taha TA, El-Nouty FD, El-Mahdy AR, Salem MH. Reproductive toxicologic effects of gossypol on male rabbits: biochemical, enzymatic, and electrolyticproperties of seminal plasma. *Fertil Steril.* 89, 2008, 1585-1593.

Smith H. *Lectures on the kidney.* University of the Kansas Press, 1943.

Stoner, G D, Mukhtar, H. Polyphenols as cancer chemopreventive agents. *J Cell Biochem,* 59(22), 1995, 169–180.

Švarc-Gajić J. Naturally occurring food toxicants. In: *Nutritional insights in food safety* (Ed: Švarc-Gajić J. Novascience Publishers, New York, 2011), 39-99.

Valentão P, Fernandes E, Carvalho F, Andrade PB, Seabra RM, Bastos ML. Antioxidant Activity of *Centaurium erythraea* Infusion Evidenced by Its Superoxide Radical Scavenging and Xanthine Oxidase Inhibitory Activity. *J Agri Food Chem* 49 (7), 2001, 3476–3479.

Valenzano DR, Terzibasi E, Genade T, Cattaneo A, Domenici L, Cellerino A. Resveratrol prolongs lifespan and retards the onset of age-related markers in a short-lived vertebrate. *Curr Biol.* 16 (3), 2006, 296–300.

White JR and Pharm D. Apple Trees to Sodium Glucose Co-Transporter Inhibitors: A Review of SGLT2 Inhibition. *Clin Diabetes.* 28(1), 2010,5-10.

Wood JG, Rogina B, Lavu S, Howitz K, Helfand SL, Tatar M, Sinclair D. Sirtuin activators mimic caloric restriction and delay ageing in metazoans. *Nature* 430 (7000), 2004, 686–289.

Wojdyło, A, Oszmiański, J, Czemerys, R. Antioxidant activity and phenolic compounds in 32 selected herbs. *Food Chem,* 1005, 2007, 940-949.

Yu C, Shin YG, Chow A, Li Y, Kosmeder JW, Lee YS, Hirschelman WH, Pezzuto JM, Mehta RG, van Breemen RB. Human, rat, and mouse metabolism of resveratrol. *Pharm Res.* 19(12), 2002, 1907-1914.

Yoon, JH, Baek, SJ. Molecular targets of dietary polyphenols with anti-inflammatory properties. *Yonsei Med J,* 46, 2006, 585-595.

Zhu PD. Electron microscopic observations on the effects of gossypol on the human endometrium. *Zhonghua Fu Chan Ke Za Zhi* 19, 1984, 246-258.

Chapter VI

RISKS ASSOCIATED WITH BIOACTIVE FOOD INGREDIENTS

Bioactive compounds that can be found in food can be naturally produced or can be introduced via technological production processes or by other anthropogenic factors. In addition, unexpected or unknown processes, such as microbial activity, can introduce dangerous bioactive components into food. Food components have different origin and in human diet food components of plant, animal and microbial origin are represented, and some higher fungi are used in the diet as well. The food of animal origin includes animal products, such as milk and eggs, or edible tissues, like meat. These products most often carry a risk due to distribution of anthropogenic contaminants to edible parts and due to excretion of some toxins ingested via feed, or introduced through water or air. Heavy metals and persistent organic pollutants, for example, are known to be accumulated in milk, as well as mycotoxins metabolites. Mycotoxins are not by their origin anthropogenic, but are rather the reflectance of unknown, unanticipated microbial activity, or poor hygienic veterinary practice. As a result of agricultural and veterinary practice pesticide residues and veterinary drug residues can be distributed to edible animal parts. Plants and fungi produce numerous, chemically diverse bioactive compounds by themselves, which may demonstrate both beneficial and adverse effects in humans.

Bioactive food components fall into different chemical classes and have different mode of action. The effects can be demonstrated as an impairment of specific organs and systems, such as in the case of photosensitizing agents which affect skin, or hemagglutinins which provoke blood agglutination, or may have systematic effects by binding to hormone receptors or affecting nervous system. Some food bioactive components exhibit high acute toxicity, like cyanogenic glycosides, whereas others are dangerous for their carcinogenic, procarcinogenic or teratogenic effects.

1. BIOGENIC AMINES

Bioactive amines, like adrenaline, dopamine, agmantine, phenylethylamine, serotonin and others, may be synthetized by some plants, like bananas, pineapple and avocado, at moderate doses. The content of several biogenic amines is particularly high in processed or fermented food like wine, cheese, cured meat, fish, pickled vegetables, chocolate, fermented sauces, where they are produced by microbial activity from free amino acids (Figure VI.1). Free amino acids are released as a result of proteolytic activity on food proteins. Produced amines are physiologically active, but are not acutely very toxic (Table VI.1). In most of cases their effects are insignificant because humans have developed an enzymatic system involving monoamine oxidase (MAO), diamine oxidase and histamine-N- methyltransferase to inactivate them. Sensitive individuals, however, or those receiving antidepressant therapies implying MAO inhibitors, may develop severe reactions.

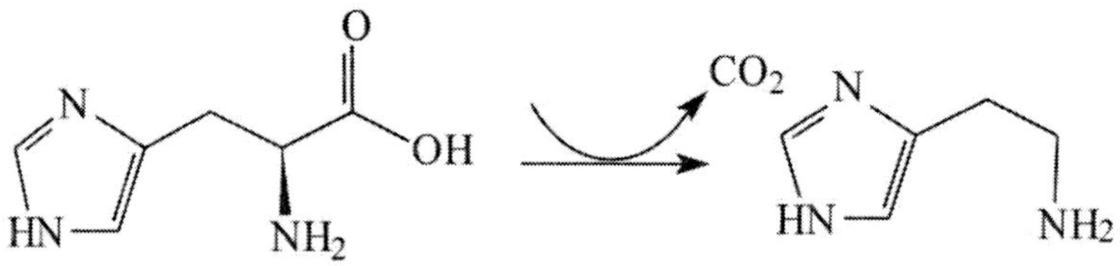

Figure VI.1. The production of histamine from histidin.

Amines produced in food negatively influence sensory properties. Tyramine indicates aging of food products while cadaverine and putrescine indicate food spoilage. These amines are also formed during putrefaction of animal tissue. In plants they bind to pectin delaying fruit softening. Polyamines spermidine, spermine and putrescine, are normally found in human fluids and are responsible for the distinctive odor of urine and semen. In their protonated form they interact with negatively charged DNA and phospholipids (Švarc-Gajić, 2011).

Table VI.1. Acute toxicity of bioactive amines

Amine	Precursor amino acid	Acute toxicity (LD_{50}) (rats, oral)
Tyramine	Tyrosine	710 mg/kg (mouse, intraperitoneal)
Histamine	Histidine	807 mg/kg (mouse, oral)
Cadaverine	Lysine	>2000 mg/kg (rat, oral)
Putrescine	L-ornithine	2000 mg/kg (rat/oral)
Spermidine	Methionine Arginine	600 mg/kg (rat/oral)
Spermine	Methionine Arginine	600 mg/kg (rat/oral)

Biogenic amines, like adrenaline, noradrenalin, histamine, serotonin and tryptamin, have a complex role in human body. Sensitive individuals with low enzyme activity or individuals receiving MAO therapy can develop apparent intolerance to specific food high in amines. Intolerance is demonstrated through headaches, flushing, hives and asthma attacks. Headache results from selective cerebral vasoconstriction. In severe cases even anaphylactic shock may occur. Apparent tolerance to dietary food amines may be developed. Ingested through food, amines are not able to pass blood/brain barrier, however they provoke release of stored endogenous biogenic amines. With repeated exposures stored amines are depleted reducing the severity of symptoms.

2. AMINO-ACID ANALOGS

Analogs of amino acids are numerous in nature (Table VI.2). Representing primary plant metabolites, many of them are biologically active.

Large brown beans, *Archidendron pauciflorum* (*Pitchecellobium jiringa, Pitchecellobium lobatum, Archidendron jiringa*), are consumed in Southeast Asia – Malaysia, Indonesia, Thailand, in typical dishes like curry and satay. When not detoxified the beans can cause poisoning due to sulphur-containing non–protein amino acid called *djenkolic acid* (Figure VI.2). The content of djenkol in the seeds is normally in the range 0.3-1.3%. The risk of adverse effects of djenkol is reduced by boiling the beans prior preparing meals.

Table VI.2. Natural analogs of amino acids.

Protein amino acids	Structurally related plant amino acids
Arginine	Canavanine
Glutamic acid	β-N-methylaminoalanine (BMAA)
Leucine	Leucine hydroxides (e.g. 5-hydroxyleucine)
Phenylalanine	m-Tyrosine, o-tyrosine
Proline	Azetidine, proline hydroxides (e.g. *trans*-3-hydroxyproline, *trans*-4-hydroxyproline)
Tyrosine	3,4-Dihydroxyphenylalanine (DOPA)
Valine	Valine hydroxides (e.g. 4-hydroxyvaline)

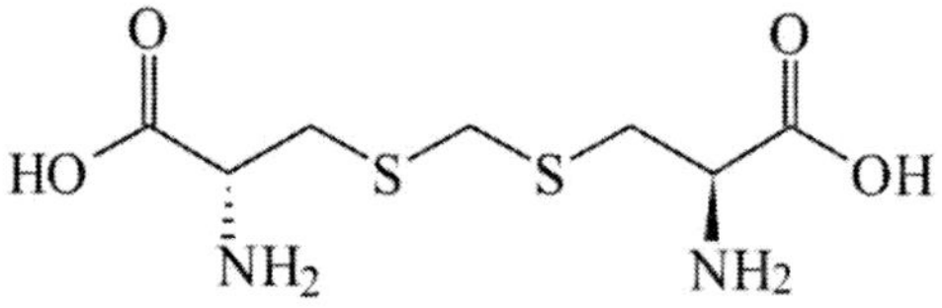

Figure VI.2. Djenkol.

After ingestion djenkol crystallizes in urinary tract and mechanically damages renal tubules provoking severe colic's, hematuria, nausea and vomiting (Švarc-Gajić, 2011).

In cases of severe poisoning needles-like crystals of djenkol can be seen in urine. Symptoms appear several hours upon ingestion. In poisoning cases it is useful to administrate sodium bicarbonate and to increase water intake in order to accelerate dissolution of the toxic acid.

Hypoglycine (Figure VI.3) is found in Jamaican fruit (*Blighia sapida*), also called ackee or akee. The fruit originates from West Africa and was brought to Jamaica in the 18th century. The fruit contains two types of hypoglycine, A and B. Hypoglycine A is found in both seeds and arils of the plant, while hypoglycine B is found only in seeds. Unripened fruit has the highest content of this toxic amino acids, structurally similar to lysine. Levels of hypoglycine A in ackee arils peak at maturity but rapidly diminish to non-detectable levels in opened fruit making it safe for consumption. In Jamaica the harvesting techniques of ackee are improved and optimized so today cases of poisoning with hypoglycine are rare.

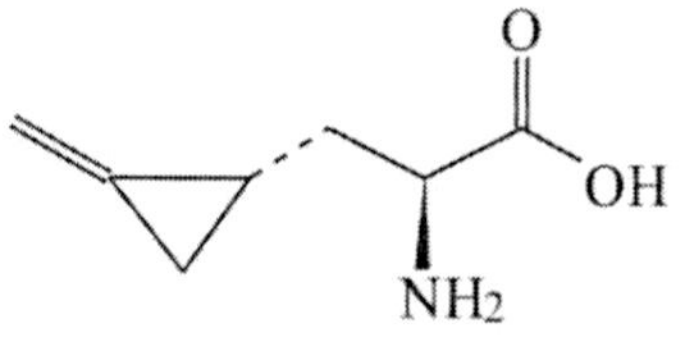

Figure VI.3. Hypoglycine A.

The toxicity of hypoglycine arises from competitive binding to enzymes involved in fatty acid metabolism, more particularly carnitine acyltransferases and acyl-CoA dehydrogenase, as well as irreversible binding to coenzyme A and carnitine I. By affecting metabolic enzymes involved in beta oxidation of fatty acids, hypoglycines reduce their bioavailability. Beta oxidation is important and is closely linked to glycolysis, both providing body with ATP, NADH, and acetyl CoA. Due to perturbed beta oxidation glucose metabolism is used to produce energy and acetyl CoA in cell mitochondria. As a result hypoglycemia develops, accompanied with lethargy and unconsciousness. First symptoms, like nausea and vomiting, appear 2-3h upon ingestion (Švarc-Gajić, 2011). Instead of beta oxidation of fatty acids omega oxidation takes place in endoplasmatic reticulum. As a major metabolic product dicarboxylic acid is produced, this is eliminated by urinary tract and may serve as a reliable indicator of poisoning with ackee fruit.

Lathyrogens are derivatives of amino acids found in legumes used in human and animal diet, like chick peas, vetch, sweat pea, grass pea and other. When consumed row, these legumes can cause serious risk to humans and grazing animals. Poisoning with lathyrogens is denoted as lathyrism and is frequent in India, China and some parts of Mediterranean. Two types of lathyrism can be recognized, depending on whether nervous system, or bones and connective tissue are attacked. Poisoning with affected nervous or bone and connective tissue systems are known as neurolathyrism and osteolathyrism, respectively.

Neurolathyrism occurs as a result of antagonism with glutamic acid by neurolathyrogens. Glutamic acid is an important neurotransmitter. The effects of neurolathyrogens can be irreversible due to damage to mitochondria in motor neurons which causes cell death (Švarc-Gajić, 2011). Neurolathyrism is demonstrated as loss of strength in lower limbs and irreversible paralysis. The symptoms of osteolathyrism, like loosening of connective tissue, tinning of bones and bone deformities, are also likely to be irreversible. Lathyrogens like β-aminopropionitrile inhibit copper-containing enzyme lysil oxidase responsible for cross-linking of procollagen and proelastin in connective tissue and built-up of strong covalent cross-links between collagen tertiary structures in bones.

Selenoamino acids are selenium-containing amino acids structurally similar to sulphur-containing amino acids. Biochemical paths of functional sulphur-containing amino acids and selenoamino acids are very similar and selenium excess may cause the production of different non-functional proteins. Selenium is essential element which is incorporated in numerous enzymes involved in iodine metabolism, immune response and protection from harmful peroxides. High doses of the element, however, are extremely toxic. First evidence of selenium toxicity was reported when Marco Polo visited China in 13th century. Horses which grazed on selenium high plants developed severe symptoms, like stiff gait and loosening of hooves. Selenium content in plants primarily depends on soil selenium, and some World regions, like United States, China, Ireland, Australia and Israel, are known to have elevated selenium concentrations. Selenium accumulators (*Oonopsis, Xylorrhiza, Astragalus* spp.) grow only on selenium-rich soils and may accumulate up to 15, 000 ppm of the element. In such plants most of selenium is not incorporated in proteins but is in the form of free amino acids like Se-methyl-selenocysteine. Secondary selenium absorbers (*Aster, Atriplex* spp.) accumulate the element in amount of several hundreds of ppm only if they grow on seleniferous soil, but they can equally well grow on a soil containing average selenium contents posing a risk to humans and animals only if soil on which they are grown is selenium rich.

Acute poisoning with selenium is characterized by nausea, dizziness, vomiting and loss of hair and nails (Švarc-Gajić, 2011). In prolonged exposures skin discoloration and dental caries can develop.

Monkeys' coconut (*Lecithin ollaria*) grows in Venezuela and Brazil and is related to Brazil nut (*Bertholletia excelsa*). Both trees produce woody, thick-walled seed capsules about a size of a large grapefruit. The toxic component of these selenium-accumulating plants is seleno-cystathionine. Selenium content in tasteful nuts is so high that death cases in children after consuming only several nuts were reported.

3. BIOACTIVE COMPOUNDS FROM SPICES

Addition of *spices* to food dates far beck in the history. In the Middle Ages spices were among the most appreciated and luxurious products available in Europe. Besides giving food specific flavor and enhancing sensory properties, spices were added to food as a mean of preservation. Strong antimicrobial properties of spices extended the shelf life of food products when other means of food preservation were unavailable. Spice plants produce chemically diverse active substances and besides their use as food components, spices have a long history of being used as aphrodisiacs, stimulants and drugs in folk medicines.

Capsaicin is the principle pungent component of chili peppers, genus *Capsicum*. There are five species of Capsicum peppers, with the hottest belonging to *Capsicum chinense* group. In plants capsaicin is produced as a secondary metabolite to repel herbivores and to protect plants against fungi. Compounds chemically related to capsaicin, and also contributing to pungency, are called capsaicinoids. *Capsicum annum* contains approximately 1.27% of capsaicinoids among which 0.03% is capsaicin. Other capsaicinoids in peppersareless abundant and less pungent. According to its pungency, dihydrocapsaicine, which contributes to total capsaicinoids content significantly, is very close to capsaicin. Dilute solutions of different capsaicinoids produce different types of pungency.

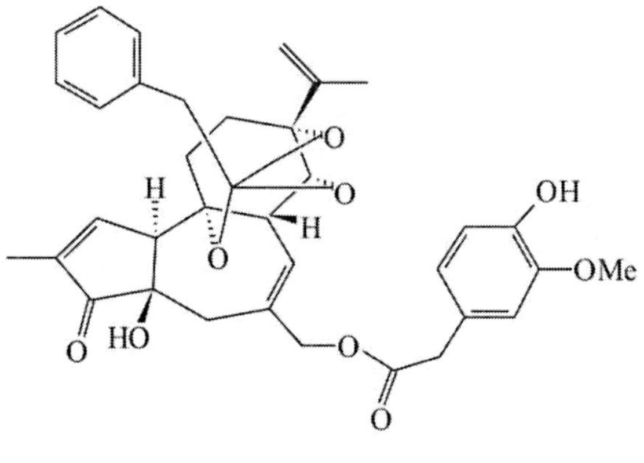

Figure VI.4. Resiniferatoxin.

Capsaicin is highest in placental tissue and internal membranes covering the seeds. The seeds themselves do not produce capsaicin and are important in plant reproduction because they are predominantly dispersed by birds which remain unaffected by capsaicin due to lack of capsaicin-responsive receptors. Pepper seeds consumed by birds pass through their digestive tract intacked and germinate later. An extremely potent natural capsaicin analogue that mimics cellular action of capsaicin, a resiniferatoxin (Figure VI.4), was found in a cactus-like plant (*Euphorbia resinifera*), commonly grown in Morocco.

Capsaicin binds to TrpV1 (Transient receptor potential cation channel subfamily V member 1) neural receptors present at both sides of plasma membranes (Dray, 1992). TrpV1 receptors are non-selective cation channels activated by heat (>43°C), low pH, physical abrasion, capsaicin and other pungent compounds. Activation of these receptors leads to painful burning sensation or abrasive-like effects. Once activated TrpV1 receptors increase permeability of membrane to cations, especially to calcium, causing the release of inflammatory mediators and signaling the pain. In prolonged activation of TrpV1 receptors an inverse effects are observed, i.e. the cessation of pain signaling. Prolonged activation of neurons depletes presynaptic neuropeptide P, one of the 100 known neurotransmitters for pain and heat. Neuropeptides are distinct from larger neurotransmitters and they modulate neuronal communication by acting on cell surface receptors.

Capsaicin is well absorbed from gastrointestinal tract (85%) and poorly through skin. After absorption the compound is rapidly distributed to other organs and is metabolized by cytochrome P450 enzymes. Peak plasma concentration is reached after 5h. IARC (International Agency for Research on Cancer) and EPA (Environmental Protection Agency) failed to classify capsaicin in respect to its carcinogenic character because of inconclusive results obtained in animal models. In some animal studies carcinogenic, procarcinogenic, cocarcinogenic, and tumor promotion effects of capsaicin were reported. However in *in vitro* studies conducted with human prostate cancer and lung cancer cells anti-proliferative effects were reported. Capsaicin also inhibited the growth of leukemic cells (Švarc-Gajić, 2011). Humans are exposed to capsaicin by ingesting chili pepper or hot food, or topically, by skin contact with chili peppers or chili products. Contact of skin and mucose membranes with capsaicin provokes heating sensation. Treatment of capsaicin effects on the skin should include cooling for burning sensation and treatment with local anesthetics. Capsaicin cannot be removed from the skin and mucose membranes by water due to its hydrophobic character, and rather a soap or detergency, hydrophobic creams or oils, should be used. In capsaicin-induced asthma bronchodilatators and antihistamines are usually administrated.

For its ability to arrest pain capsaicin is nowadays used as a topical analgesic (0.025% - 0.075%) in conditions like arthritis, diabetic neuropathy and muscle pain. Long-term loss of neural responsiveness to pain under the influence of capsaicin is related to the destruction of neural pain receptors with high doses of capsaicin. Capsaicin is also a registered insectide, miticide, rodenticide, used on crops, buildings and containers to rappel rabbits, squirrels, deer's, raccoons, cats, dogs and skunks. Due to its antimicrobial properties the compound is used as a marine antifoulant and to treat psoriasis.

Piperine is found in plants of Piperaceae family, such as black pepper (*Piper nigrum*) and long pepper (*Piper longum*) and is stored mostly in fruits where it constitutes 3 - 7%. Piperine is composed of alkaloid piperidine and piperic acid (Figure VI.5). Chavicine, a compound related to piperine, accompanies it in black pepper contributing to peppers pungency. Both pungent substances are secondary plant metabolites. Pepper was prized since antiquity for both its flavor and its antiseptic properties widely exploited in folk medicine to treat malaria, ear inflammation, gangrene and other infectious diseases. The pungency of piperine, similarly to capsaicin, is caused by activation of ion channels on pain sensing nerve cells (nociceptors). For its stronger potency in comparison to capsaicin, piperine is used as a chemical template for the design of improved TrpV1 agonists.

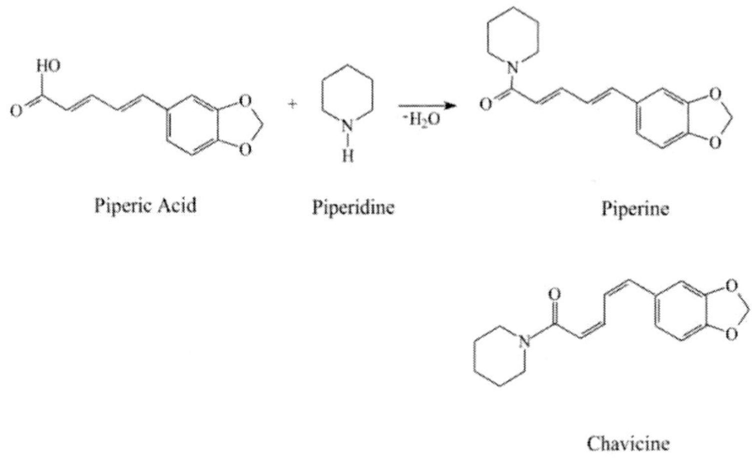

Piperic Acid   Piperidine   Piperine

Chavicine

Figure VI.5. Chemical structures of piperine and related chavicine.

In addition to antimicrobial, bactericidal and insecticidal effects, piperine demonstrates strong antioxidant, anti-inflammatory and anti-tumor potential. In rat models the compound provoked the decrease in arterial pressure in dose-dependent manner (Taqvi et al., 2008). Alcoholic extract of black pepper showed to be cytotoxic to human lymphoma cells and in mice bearing carcinoma piperine inhibited solid tumor development. Administration of black pepper extract to test animals with carcinoma prolonged the life span for 37.3% - 58.8% (Vijayan and Thampuran, 2000). Piperine has, however, demonstrated neurotoxicity to cultured neurons (Unchern et al., 1998) and interfered with reproductive events in mammalian models (Vijayan and Thampuran, 2000).

Physiologically active by itself, piperine also demonstrates several marked physiological effects indirectly by affecting metabolism of other exogenous substances due to its pronounced impact on protein transporters. Piperine affects mostly transporters in intestinal linings activating them and increasing the absorption of selenium, β-carotene, vitamins B, sparteine and other compounds (Švarc-Gajić, 2011). By the same mechanism piperine increases curcumin bioavailability by remarkable 2000% for what curcumin supplements are formulated almost exclusively in combination with piperine. On contrary to activation of gut protein transporters, piperine inhibits P protein, as well as microsomal enzymes involved in metabolism of endogenous and exogenous substances. P protein is a vital protein participating in the transport of compounds from intracellular space. Inhibited P protein indirectly prolongs the residence time of the compounds in cells potentiating their effects. Altered metabolism of the compounds due to piperine influence can significantly affect therapeutic dose of drugs. Piperine strongly interacts with metabolism of antiepileptic drug Phenytoin, non-selective beta blocker Propranolol and bactericide Rifamipicin (Rifampin). Metabolism and bioavailability of other substances may also be inhibited due to piperine effects on the production of glucuronic acid. The conjugates with glucuronic acid are important means of toxicant excretion and lack of glucuronic acid prolongs the residence time of xenobiotics in the body.

In conclusion, spices represent rich natural sources of various highly bioactive compounds, however in equilibrated diet they are not normally used in great quantities. On contrary, the intake of more common food containing bioactive compounds in some circumstances may be significant, especially in uniform diet.

4. BIOACTIVE COMPOUNDS FROM COMMON FOOD

Avocado (*Persea americana*) naturally produces persin (Figure VI.6), a fungicidal and insecticidal substance which has been shown to trigger allergic reactions in humans (Blanko et al., 1994). Persin was identified only recently, revealing that chemical structure is similar to linoleic acid. Earlier it was considered that toxic chemical was restricted to leaves, bark, pits and skin of avocado tree. However, the literature has reported adverse effects after fruit consumption in both humans and animals (Blanko et al., 1994, Buoro et al., 1994). In Mexico, after detoxification by steaming, the leaves of avocado are used for preparing some typical dishes.

First evidenced toxicity of persin was demonstrated in silk worms and fungi, and later on in birds and mammals. Persin may represent a serious risk to domestic animals causing non-infectious mastitis and agalactia, gastrointestinal distress and anaphylaxis (Švarc-Gajić, 2011). In acute overdoses with persin, above 100 mg/kg, throat and chest edema is experienced and death arises due to heart arrest. Histopathological tests show microscopically extensive death of heart cells, as well as necrosis of myocardial fibers (Grant et al., 1991).

Today persin attracts attention of scientists because it was discovered that it acts synergistically with breast cancer drugs, binding to steroid hormone receptors and modulating their responsiveness to the drugs (Švarc-Gajić, 2011). The effects of persin make breast cancer cells more susceptible to breast cancer drugs.

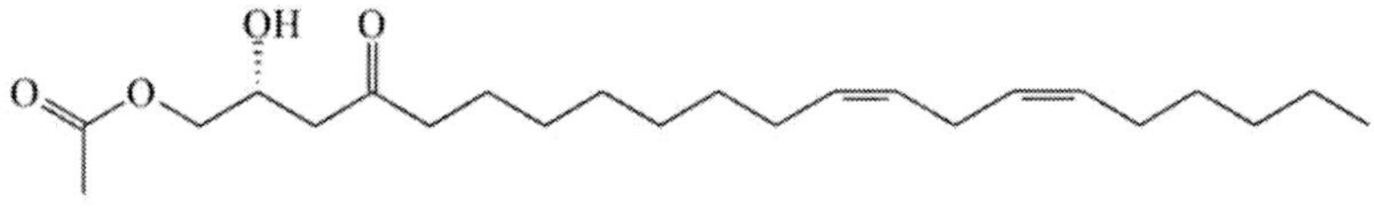

Figure VI.6. Persin.

Finger cherry (*Rhodomyrtus macrocarpa*) is indigenous Australian plant that produces elongated, finger-like fruits. Small hairy tree grows in rainforests. The consumption of attractive fruit by Aborigines and animals was linked to numerous cases of permanent blindness in livestock and children. Even though exact mechanism of toxic action is unknown it is speculated that toxic dibenzofurans, called rhodomyrtoxins, in combination with some saponins that plant produces, are responsible for such effects (Švarc-Gajić,

2011). After the toxicity of the finger cherry has been recognized the fruit was banned for the consumption by Australian authorities, however Aborigines continue to consume this fruit, sometimes without any toxic effects. According to one theory a fungus, growing on a tree, is, in fact, responsible for toxin production.

Miracle fruit (*Synsepalum dulcificum*) grows in tropics and produces berries which, when consumed, alter the responsiveness of taste receptors rendering sour food like lime and lemon, sweet. A fruit glycoprotein, miraculin, binds to taste buds and changes the shape of sweetness receptors, making them responsive to acids (Švarc-Gajić, 2011). The effects of miraculin last about half an hour. The fruit itself has a very subtle sweet taste. Curculin from *Malaysian fruit* (*Curculigo latifolia*) and thaumatins from West Africa *Katemfe fruit* (*Thaumatococcus daniellii*) produce similar effects. All glycoproteins are heat sensitive and lose their effects upon heating. Curculin itself has a sweet taste up to several hundreds to thousand times stronger than sucrose. Thaumatins, which are a mixture of different proteins, also have pronounced sweet taste, up to 2000 times stronger in comparison to sucrose, as well as flavor modifying properties. Sweet taste of miraculin, curculin and thaumatins, is build-up gradually and lasts longer in comparison to sucrose, leaving a sweet aftertaste.

Miraculin was considered as a low-calorie sweetener but was prevented by FDA which classified miraculin as a food additive. Nowadays miraculin is sold in the form of tablets, granules, and candies, and is available as a commercial product used for fun. If precaution is not taken the use of miraculin-based fun products may cause the development of stomach ulcers due to overconsumption of very acidic or hot food, like chili, pickles, limes, peppers etc., which become completely masked due to altered taste signals.

The *Olive tree* is native to Palestine. Its leaves and oil were used since the antiquity for different purposes, to mummify dad and to prepare medicines. Olive tree produces a myriad of bioactive compounds, such as beta-carotene, phytosterols, flavonoids luteolin and quercetin, as well as other phenolic compounds. Phenolic compounds, predominantly oleuropein and tyrosol, are responsible for bitter and pungent taste of the olive oil, but also for its potent antioxidant capacity. Olive oil is high in oleic acid (Figure VI.7), a monounsaturated omega-9 fatty acid. In glyceride form this acid makes up to 80%. Free oleic acid in oil originates from the breakdown of triacylglycerydes. Olive oil is thus, classified according to free acid content, measured as free oleic acid, to extra virgin (1% of free oleic acid), virgin (2% of free oleic acid) and ordinary (3.3% of free oleic acid). Unrefined olive oil contains more than 3.3% of free oleic acid and is considered unfit for human consumption.

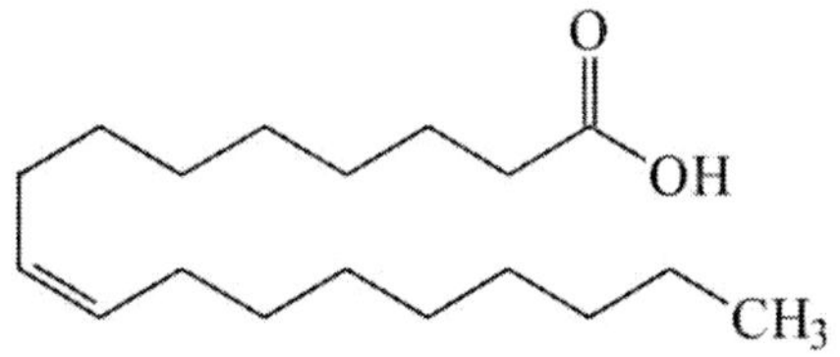

Figure VI.7. Oleic acid, a monounsaturated omega-9 fatty acid.

Due to high content of phenols olive oil has strong antioxidant and anti-inflammatory effects. It is believed that one spoon of the oil has stronger antioxidant potential than a glass of red wine, and that 50 g of the olive oil is equivalent to 0.1 g of ibuprofen (Beauchamp et al., 2005). Olive oil mixed with ozone is promoted for insect stings and bites, as well as for bacterial and fungal skin infections. For constipation it is recommended to take 30 ml of the olive oil in a single dose because the oil improves peristalsis and boosts gut bacteria. Due to high content of squalene olive oil can be used as a shaving lubricant, hair tonic, to exfoliate hands and face and to treat stretch marks.

Oleuropein (Figure VI.8), a glucoside found in leaves, bark, root and fruit, makes the olive plant highly resistant to insect damage and other diseases. Oleuropein and hydoxytyrosol are two principal and most bioactive phenolic compounds. Antioxidant capacity of oleuropein is greater in comparison to phenols in green tea and about 400 times stronger in comparison to vitamin C (Visioli et al., 2000). For isolation of oleuropein leaves of the olive tree are used. Oleuropein preparations are available in the form of liquid concentrates, dried olive leaves, powder and capsules.

Oleuropein supplements are not recommended in persons suffering from low blood pressure and glucose, because the compound radically lowers blood pressure and plasma glucose. Consequently these supplements should not be combined with drugs for regulating diabetes. If taken on empty stomach supplements may provoke stomach discomfort and temporary loss of appetite. Due to high antimicrobial activity and detoxifying reactions undergoing in liver, kidneys and intestines, resulting in overburden with phagocyted microbial cells, upon supplements ingestion flu-like symptoms may be experienced.

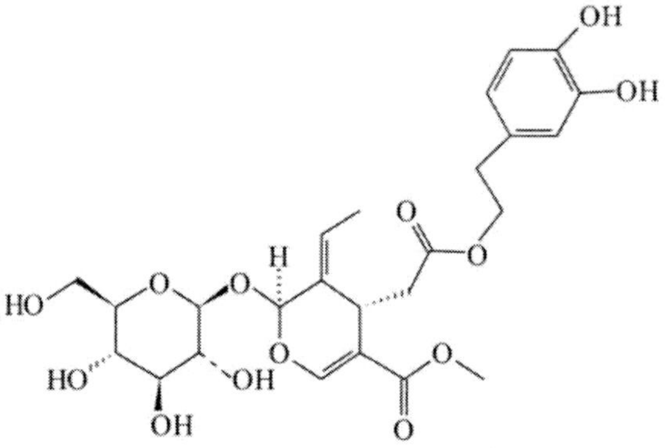

Figure VI.8. Oleuropein, a principal phenolic compound in olives.

Papaya (*Carica papaya*) is native to tropics and was first cultivated in Mexico. The fruit is susceptible to papaya ringspot virus, which causes deformation of leaves, as well as to fruit fly which lays its eggs in young fruits. The black seeds of papaya are edible as well and are used as a cheaper substitution to black pepper due to their sharp, pungent and spicy taste. In some parts of Asia, young leaves of papaya are steamed and prepared like spinach dishes.

The pungency of papaya seeds originates from isothio-compound, similar to those of cauliflower and cabbage that are formed by mirosinaze transformation of thioglucoside (Figure 8). Formed benzyl-isothycyanate induces glutathione-S-transferase, an enzyme important for detoxification of xenobiotics.

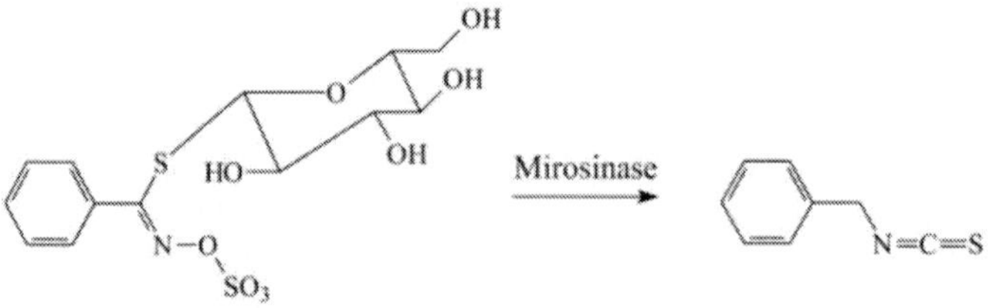

Glucotrapaedin   Benzyl-isothiocyanate

Figure VI.9. Enzymatically catalyzed formation of pungent benzyl-isothiocyanate in papaya.

Green papaya fruit and tree latex are rich in proteolytic enzymes papain, chymopapains A and B, papaya peptidase A, chinitases, protease inhibitors and linamarase (Krishna et al., 2008). These enzymes, highly concentrated in the plants sap, are responsible for irritating properties of unripened fruits. As fruit ripens, papain and less potent chymopapain diminish and neither is present in ripe fruit. Proteolytic potency of papain is used in cosmetics to smoothen the skin and to treat cuts, rashes, stings and burns. Isolated papain is sold in powdered or tablet form and is also used as a meat tenderizer or for enzyme therapy in gluten intolerance, as well as a digestive aid. Other proteins with unknown function have also been discovered in papaya. In papaya leaves other bioactive components, namely flavonoids, saponins, tannins, cardiac glycosides and antraquinones, have been identified.

Due to effects of benzyl isothiocyanate ground air-dried papaya seeds in dose 3 g of seeds/kg bodyweight are used in veterinary practice as anthelmintics.

Papain has the ability to dissolve dead tissue without damaging living cells for what it is used to treat ulcers, burns and scars. Chymopapain has also been used to aid in healing and recovery of surgical wounds. In folk medicine indigenous to Central America instead of isolated enzymes crushed seeds or slices of unripe fruit are used. Anti-hypertensive effects of papaya fruit, which cause decrease in systolic, diastolic, and mean arterial blood pressure, are speculated to be attributed to alkaloid carpaine (Figure VI.10) or to yet unidentified compound for which it is known to bind to alpha-adrenoreceptors (Burdick, 1971). The effects of carpaine may be related to its macrocyclic dilactone structure, and possible cation chelating effect. Fresh papaya juice lowers serum cholesterol and triglycerides. In folk medicine of the Indian subcontinent, green papaya and seed extract were used as contraception and for performing abortion. Abortifacient effect of papaya is believed to occur due to proteolytic activity that dissolves proteins responsible for adhesion of newly fertilized egg to walls of the uterus. In addition, it is known that papain suppresses progesterone (Krishna et al., 2008).

Consumption of unripe papaya can cause uterine contractions and changes in blood clothing ability. Inhalation of papaya powder can induce allergies and irritating reactions and damage to lung alveoli. Effects in respiratory tract are partially caused by high concentrations of cyanogenic glucosides which release toxic cyanide upon inhalation. Cyanogenic glucosides are particularly high in leaves and roots of the papaya tree. In animal studies conducted with crude papain some teratogenic and embryotoxic effects were demonstrated. In rabbits and rats crude papain acted as promoter and accelerated the appearance of liver tumors induced by liver carcinogen. Overconsumption of ripe papaya can cause carotenodermia, a yellow discoloration especially expressed in soles and palms, occurring due to high content (~6%) of beta carotene which upon ingestion accumulates in the skin.

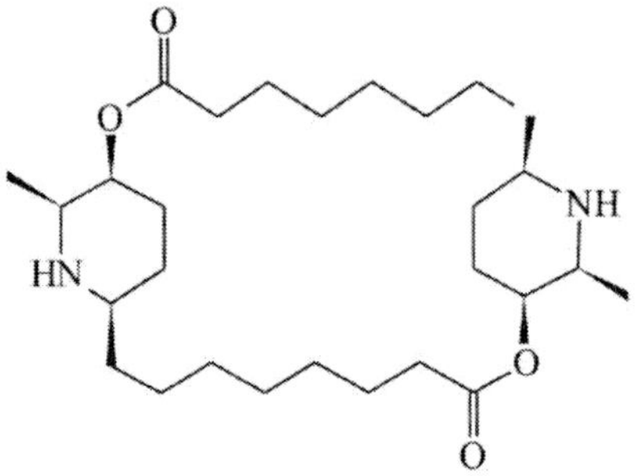

Figure VI.10. Carpaine, a macrocyclic alkaloid found in papaya fruit.

It can be said that **wine** consumption has become a cult all over the World. To many consumers appreciating tradition, history and art of wine production, wine represents far more than just a beverage. Cultural habit of wine drinking, besides enjoying in its rich taste, is also linked to beneficial health effects and one glass of wine is strongly recommended by medical personnel to prevent cardiovascular diseases. This beverage of extremely complex composition, however, in sensitive individuals may cause some adverse effects. Wine is high in organic acids like acetic, malic and tartaric that may contribute to wearing of the tooth enamel exposing dentine. Exposed dentine increases the prevalence of tooth decay and provokes sensibility to cold, hot, sweet and acidic food. Sulfites occur naturally in all wines to some extent, but are also commonly introduced to wines to stop fermentation or as a preservative. In sensitive individuals sulfites may trigger allergic reactions and it has been shown that individuals suffering from asthma are particularly sensitive and prone to sulfite-induced allergies. Common symptoms of allergic reactions include migraines, hives, nausea and in very severe cases even anaphylactic shock may occur. Similar symptoms may, however, also be caused by high histamine content. Wine, as a fermented beverage, is high in biogenic amines that in individuals with low MAO enzymatic activity cause similar effects. Red wines are high in tannins that have been shown in animal studies to decrease feed intake and feed efficiency due to chelating properties to essential minerals, especially iron (Brune et al., 1998). The bioavailability of chelated iron reduces remarkably, increasing the risk of anemia and mineral deficiency. In experiments conducted with pure tannins increase in the incidence of esophageal cancer was noted (Lewis et al., 1977). The effects depended on dosage and type of tannins. In experiments with rats in two-year study dosages of 0.25% and 0.5% caused the development of variety of tumors (Onodera et al., 1994).

REFERENCES

Beauchamp GK, Keast RSJ, Morel D, Lin J, Pika J, Han Q, Lee CH, Smith AB, Breslin, PAS. Ibuprofen-like activity in extra-virgin olive oil. *Nature*, 437, 2005,45-46.

Blanco C, Carrillo T, Castillo R, Quiralte J, Cuevas M. Avocado hypersensitivity. *Allergy* 49(6), 1994, 454-459.

Brune M, Rossander L, Hallberg L. Iron absorption and phenolic compounds: importance of different phenolic structures. *Eur J Clin Nutr* 43 (8), 1998, 547–557.

Buoro IB, Nyamwange SB, Chai D, Munyua SM. Putative avocado toxicity in two dogs. *Onderstepoort J Vet Res.* 61(1), 1994, 107–109.

Burdick EM. Carpaine: An Alkaloid of Carica Papaya: Its Chemistry and Pharmacology. *Economic Botany* 25(4), 1971, 363-365.

Dray A. Mechanism of action of capsaicin-like molecules on sensory neurons. *Life Sci.* 51 (23), 1992, 1759–1765.

Grant R., Basson PA, Booker HH, Hofherr JB, Anthonissen M. Cardiomyopathy caused by avocado (*Persea americana* Mill) *J S Afr Assoc* 62(1), 1991, 21-22.

Krishna KL, Paridhavi JA, Patel JA. Review on nutritional, medicinal and pharmacological properties of Papaya (*Carica papaya* Linn.). *Natural Prod Rad* 7(4), 2008, 364-373.

Lewis E, Memory PF, Lewis, A, Hepworth, W. *Medical botany: plants affecting man's health.* New York, Wiley, 1977.

Onodera H, Kitaura K, Mitsumori K, Yoshida J, Yasuhara K, Shimo T, Takahashi M, Hayashi Y. Study on the carcinogenicity of tannic acid in F344 rats. *Food Chem Tox.* 32(12), 1994, 1101-1106.

Švarc-Gajić J. Naturally occurring food toxicants. In: *Nutritional insights in food safety* (Ed: Švarc-Gajić J. Nova Science Publishers, New York, 2011), 39-99.

Taqvi SI, Shah AJ, Gilani AH. Blood pressure lowering and vasomodulator effects of piperine. *J Card Pharm* 52(5), 2008, 452-458.

Unchern S, Saito H, Nishiyama N. Death of Cerebellar Granule Neurons Induced by Piperine is Distinct from that Induced by Low Potassium Medium. *Neurochem Res* 23(1), 1998, 97-102.

Vijayan KK and Thampuran RVA.Pharmacology, Toxicology and Clinical Applications of Black Pepper. In: *Black pepper (Piper nigrum L.)* (Ed: Ravindran PN) Harwood Academic Publishers, United States, 2000, 455-466.

Visioli F, Poli A, Galli C. Antioxidant and other biological activities of phenols from olives and olive oil. *Med Res Rev.* 22, 2002, 65–75.

Chapter VII

MEDICINAL USE OF VENOMS

Venoms were created naturally about 60 million years ago in order to provide defensive mechanism. Since their early appearance molecular structure of venoms has been changing and evolving simultaneously with the evolution of venom-producing organisms. Venom-producing animals are numerous and are responsible for many fatality cases around the World. Only from cone snail stings annually die about 30 people, 20 from spider bites and in matter of thousands from snake bites. Even being a cause of human fatalities, venoms today represent valuable sources of medicinally important chemicals. Modern science is oriented towards exploitation of venoms in medical purposes.

Science that studies the occurrence, toxicity and poisoning treatments related to venoms is known as *toxinology*, which is not to be confused with toxicology. Toxinology deals with chemistry of venoms, mode of venoms action and biology of venom-producing organisms. This scientific discipline also studies the structure and function of venom apparatus. Broad definition would explain toxinology as a scientific discipline dealing with microbial, plant and animal toxins, poisons and venoms.

Venoms have long been used in homeopathic remedies, however it was not until the late 19th century that venoms were scientifically investigated as medicinal compounds. In modern medicine venoms are used as therapeutic or diagnostic agents, mostly for blood disorders and relief of severe pain. Furthermore, these bioactive molecules are valuable as drug templates for creating drugs with advanced pharmacological properties.

Venoms classification is not straightforward and multiple criteria can be applied in this respect. Several criteria are mostly used:

- According to producing species (amphibians, insects, marine organisms, scorpions, snakes, etc.)
- According to mechanism of action (hematoxic, neurotoxic, cardiotoxic, etc.)
- According to chemical structure (alkaloids, terpens, lactones, peptides, etc.)

Many venoms act by neurotoxic mechanism. Neurotoxic substances attack central nervous system and affect movement, breathing, swallowing, speech and sight. Venoms also often affect cardiovascular system perturbing blood clotting (hematoxic) and affecting blood vessels and causing bleeding (hemorrhagic). Cytotoxic venoms cause very painful envenomation attacking cells or tissues and causing cell lysis. Myotoxic venoms attack muscles, whereas cardiotoxic have specific affinity to heart muscle causing death via heart failure.

Neurotoxic venoms, common to different organisms, hinder the operation of muscles and respiratory system. The venoms exhibit antagonistic or agonistic action on ion channels or acetylcholine receptors in synapses. In respect to their effects on ion channels, venoms mostly act agonistically on calcium channels or affect sodium flux that is essential for membrane depolarization. Another mechanism of neurotoxic action is the prevention of neurotransmitters function inducing paralysis. Venoms affect nicotinic or muscarinic acetylcholine receptors. Nicotinic receptors are found primarily at neuromuscular junctions while muscarinic are found mostly in central nervous system. Binding of acetylcholine to nicotinic receptors causes a conformational change resulting in the formation of pore permeable to ions. This produces a rapid increase in cellular permeability to sodium and calcium ions, depolarization and excitation, resulting in muscular contraction. Ligands binding to muscarinic receptors cause conformational change that mediates activation of intracellular G-protein. This G-protein after dissociating to subunits triggers series of intracellular events mostly via enzymatic activity.

1. SNAKE VENOMS

It is estimated that envenomation with *snake venoms* causes approximately 20,000 death cases annually around the World. Venom-producing glands in snakes were developed in early stage of evolution. The development of fangs, on the other hand, represents evolutionary improvement that enabled more efficient venom delivery. Snakes have potent, complex venoms that are in some cases produced in significant quantities, however the delivery mechanism is not always very efficient. Therefore it is important to recognize that the risk of envenomation with snake venoms is the complex function of venom potency, complexity, produced quantity and effectiveness of the delivery mechanism. Consequently even less toxic venom may represent a serious risk if it is delivered to victim in great quantity.

Great number of snake venoms have profound effects on blood coagulation. Blood homeostasis is very important for preventing clotting away from the site of a wound and avoiding thrombus formation. Blood thinning, on the other hand, can cause internal bleeding. Coagulation process responsible for blood homeostasis involves a complex set of protease reactions involving roughly 30 different proteins (Figure VIII.1). The final result of these reactions is to convert fibrinogen, a soluble protein, to insoluble strands of fibrin.

Coagulation is initiated either by intrinsic or extrinsic factors. Coagulation factors, which are circulating in their inactive forms, denoted as zymogens, are further activated. In Figure VII.1 activated forms are labeled with the lower case a. In final stages of coagulation process thrombin is activated and fibrinogen is converted to fibrin, which forms a mesh-like structure capturing platelets, other blood elements and forming a blood coagulate that prevents bleeding.

Clotting process may be impaired by inappropriate activation of clotting factors, prevention of activation or by other mechanisms. Consequently the same effect may be produced by different mechanisms allowing for the selective use of venoms to address a specific deficiency in blood chemistry. Snake venoms disturb coagulation process by three major mechanisms (Figure VII.1). Group I snake venoms activate factor X, which is of greatest importance in coagulation cascade because it converges extrinsic and intrinsic coagulation pathways further leading them through a common pathway. Group II snake venoms activate prothrombin to thrombin, whereas group III snake venoms initiate conversion of fibrinogen to fibrin, acting as thrombin-like enzymes.

In envenomation with snake venoms antivenoms should be administrated, however only one in ten cases requires antivenom due to, usually, small quantities of injected toxins. For selecting adequate antivenom detection kits are available, or, alternatively polyvalent antivenom, that is effective against venoms of several species, can be applied. In antivenom therapy there is a great risk of developing severe allergic reactions, therefore antivenoms should

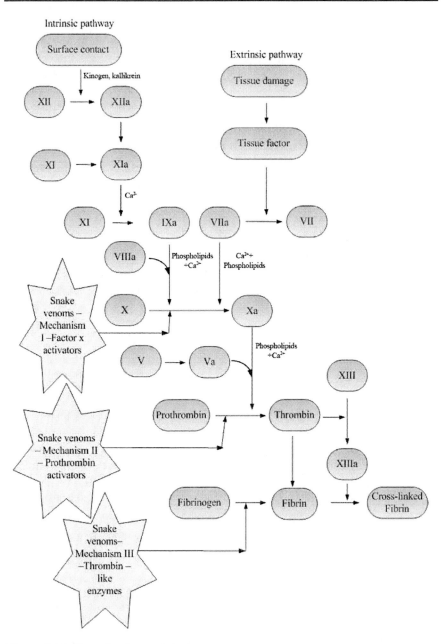

Figure VII.1. Cascade of coagulation process.

not be administrated unless there is an evidence of systematic poisoning. If the only demonstrated envenomation symptom is moderate local pain, antivenom is not indicated. Stored antivenom should never be frozen, because it loses its activity. Ampoules with venoms should be kept in refrigerator under 2-8°C protected from light. It is not rare case that efficiency of administrated antivenom varies due to natural variations in produced venoms. In envenomation treatment besides antivenom therapy adrenaline is administrated by subcutaneous route. Antihistamine, administrated parenterally, may affect sedatory and cause hypotension. To avoid allergic reaction normally prednisolone, a glucocorticoid, is given to patients for five days (Fry, 2003).

Russell's viper (*Daboia russelli*) lives in South East Asia, reaching approximately 1-1.5 meters in the length. The snake is highly venomous, causing about 6,000 deaths a year. The venom of Russell's viper activates factors V, X, IX, and protein C causing blood coagulation. Coagulative properties of snake venoms were earlier exploited in the treatment of hemophilia. The venom for this purpose is no longer used, but is a valuable diagnostic agent for detecting deficiency in clotting factor X.

Ecarin, a metalloprotease, isolated from *Echis carinatus*, is used in the analysis of blood from patients with liver diseases or patients undergoing anticoagulant therapy. The snake is found in parts of the Middle East and Central Asia, especially the Indian subcontinent. The size of the snake ranges between 38 and 80 cm in length. The importance of Ecarin is that the venom acts independently of any co-factor, catalyzing the conversion of intermediates of both carboxylated and acarboxylated prothrombin, with levels of acarboxylated prothrombin being abnormally present in patients with liver disease.

Central American pit viper (*Bothrops moojeni*) lives in Paraguay, Argentina and other Central American countries. The venom of the snake, Batroxobin, acts like thrombin-like enzyme initiating coagulation. The venom is used as a diagnostic agent to determine the levels of fibrinogen in plasma. Fibrinogen level is indirectly determined by measuring the levels of fibrin. This diagnostic agent is very useful because it allows diagnosis even in the presence of heparin allowing for a patient's plasma to be monitored for levels of fibrinogen even whilst undergoing heparin therapy.

Viprinex (Ancrod) is a therapeutic agent based on the venom isolated from the Malayan pit viper. The drug is used in stroke treatment and is effective even when given 6h after the stroke preventing new clots from forming, breaking down existing clots, and thinning out the blood (Marsten et al., 1966). Other medications used in stroke treatments are effective only in time window of 3h.

Contortrostatin, a disintegrin, was isolated from the venom of Copperhead snake (*Agkistrodon contortrix*). Disintegrins disrupt the function of other proteins called integrins, which are located on the cell surface. Integrins are involved in the adhesion process. Great medicinal potential of disintegrins arises from the fact that they selectively adhere to cancer cells, not affecting normal cells in the surrounding tissue. Experiments conducted with contortrostatin demonstrated that the compound reduces the growth rate of human breast cancer cells for 60-70% and reduces for approximately 90% tumor metastases (Swenson et al., 2004; Zhou et al., 2000).

Waglerin-1 was isolated from Wagler's Temple Viper (*Tropidolaemus wagleri*). The venom acts by blocking nicotinic acetylcholine receptors (McArdle et al., 2009). After the effects of the compound on neural receptors have been recognized a synthetic tripeptide that mimics the effects of the venom has been synthesized by Pentapharm, which runs a snake farm in Brazil. The compound has found its place in cosmetic anti-wrinkle products. Similarly to Botulinum toxin, the peptide paralyses muscle contractions by blocking nerve signals preventing the formation of expression lines.

2. LIZARD AND FROG VENOMS

Lizards produce venoms in glands located in the lower jaw and this is what distinguishes venomous systems in snakes and lizards, because in snakes the glands are located in the upper jaw. It is believed that only nine types of venoms are produced by venomous lizards. Lace Monitor Lizard venom shows that the active substance has dramatic effects on the victim's blood pressure and clotting, and that it provokes internal bleeding, revealing that its toxicity arises by disruption of coagulation processes. The saliva of Commodore Lizard besides containing venom, poses a health risk because it contains more than 50 different bacteria. Gila Monster (*Heloderma suspectum*) is native to southwestern United States and northern Mexico. The lizard doesn't inject the venom directly into the victim but the poison is transferred from the lizard's saliva into the open wounds. Because of such insufficiently effective mechanism, human fatalities from Gila monster bites are rare, however a bite can cause intense pain, nausea, swelling, fatigue, dizziness, and chills. The venom of Gila Monster is medicinally important because it stimulates insulin production, reducing blood glucose (Raufman et al., 1982). A drug Byetta is based on the venom of Gila monster and was approved by the FDA in 2005 for treating type 2 diabetes. The drug is well tolerated and doesn't cause mood swings.

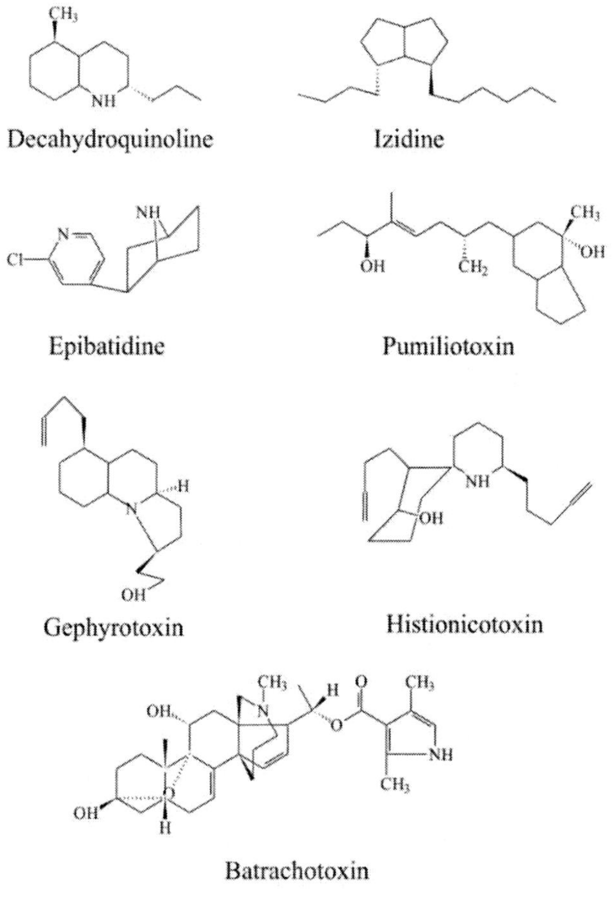

Figure VII.2. The structure of common poison arrow frog venoms.

Frog venoms were used by Amazonian tribes to tip the arrows to produce more efficient weapon. For this, poisonous frogs, mostly from Dendrobatid family, are also called poison arrow frogs. Frogs produce alkaloids through their digestive process from insects feeding on plants rich in alkaloids necessary for venom production. Produced venoms are then stored in glands just below the surface of the frog's skin and are released when the frog is threatened. Isolation of toxins from frog's skin for research and medical purposes is not always successful and is accompanied with problems of frogs loosing the ability to produce the toxins in captivity.

Frog venoms are medicinally very attractive compounds acting by different mechanisms. Pumiliotoxin (Figure VII.2) binds to sodium channels causing their opening and closing and producing persistent transmission of nerve signals which, in return, provokes uncontrollable muscle spasms. Batrachotoxin is a lipid-soluble neurotoxin that binds to sodium channels and has a huge potential as anesthetic, whereas epibatidine has a strong analgesic potency. Gephyrotoxin is a tricyclic alkaloid that blocks the passage of potassium ions and represents a tremendous interest as a potential drug.

There are more than 1700 described *scorpion* species, but only about 25 species are known to produce venom. The component of a venom of Giant Israeli scorpion (*Leiurus quinquestriatus*), a chlorotoxin, is a peptide consisting of 36 aminoacids that selectively recognizes only the cancerous cells in the brain. Advanced medicinal use of chlorotoxin implies its attachment to chemotherapeutic agent, samporin, to treat incurable form of brain cancer, glioma (Deshane et al., 2003) Another peptide, antarease, was isolated from the venom of Brazilian yellow scorpion (*Tityus serrulatus*). The peptide is used to study pancreatitis because it disrupts pancreas function.

3. INSECT VENOMS

Ants produce venoms with different bioactive components, however common to all ant colonies is the ability to repel insects, animals and birds. A bioactive component with pesticidal properties, iridomyrmecin (Figure VII.3) was first isolated from the Argentine ant. Iridomyrmecin is also found in a variety of plants. In addition to iridomyrmecin, ants produce high concentrations of insecticidal formic acid which kills feather lice and feather mites, so in the nature it can be seen that birds cover instinctively themselves with ants. Insecticidal properties of ant venoms were used by humans as well. People used to put clothing infected with lice on anthills for disinfection.

Varieties of ant species are quite vast. Some ants have a stinger, similar to a wasp, whereas others produce poisonous fluid, containing formic acid and alkaloids, which is sprayed by the insect at a distance of up to 10 cm. Nest ants, or green tree ants (*Oecophylla smaragdina*), make hard nests on the trees.

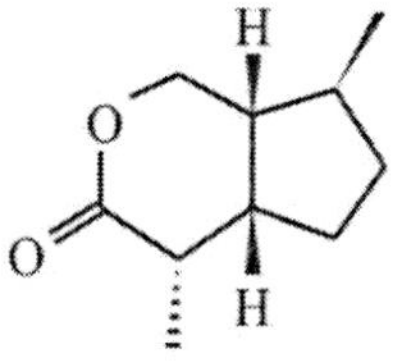

Figure VII.3. Iridomyrmecin.

Giant tropical bullet ant (*Paraponera clavata*) is considered to be the most toxic ant species. There is a ritual among some Amazonian tribes that involves intentional envenomation with the Giant tropical bullet ant. Young men seeking marriage ought to put their hands into ant nests to show that they can withstand pain and that they are ready to deal with obligations imposed by marriage. Ant envenomation is accompanied with severe pain with numbness, vomiting and uncontrollable trembling that last 24h, for what the ant is also known as "Hormiga Veinticuatro" or "24 hour ant", referring to 24 hours of pain that follows ant stings. Harvester ants (*Pogonomyrmex micans*) live in Africa and have unpleasant odor that respells insects. Touching the ants with bare hands causes inflammation, fingernails loosening and falling out. A single colony of South American leaf-cutter ant (*Atta cephalotes*) can count up to 5 million members, and each colony has one queen that can live more than 15 years. Envenomation with South American leaf-cutter ant causes painful inflammation and ulcers.

Since ants live in large colonies they evolved a defense mechanism against bacteria, viruses and fungi. Ant venom contains formic acid (50-79%), which was named after the red ant *Formica rufa*, as well as other antiseptic compounds, like phenol and phenylacetic acid. Phenol as an antiseptic is highly effective against staphylococcus bacteria and *Candida* (Veal, 1992). In addition, ant venom contains formic aldehydes, ATP and more than 19 enzymes. In Chinese medicine it is believed that formic acid increases appetite and stimulates lactation. In some species formic acid constitutes up to 20% of the total body weight in ants. In some traditional medicines small amounts of formic acid are believed to stimulate sexual desire. Due to antiseptic properties of ant venoms humans used to mix the soil surrounding ant hills with water and to use it internally for diarrhea and dysentery.

Medicinal use of ant venom dates far beck in the history. The Roman writer Plutarch described that bears suffering from abdominal complaints put their tongues into honey and then into an ant hill. When the tongue was covered with ants they swallowed them as a remedy. In the Middle Ages ant venom was taken as a tonic, stomachic, diuretic and aphrodisiac. Famous seventeenth century vinegar was made with ants and was mentioned in the London Pharmacopoeia of 1696.

Ants with biting jaws were used by Amazonian tribes to stitch up wounds, whereas other ant varieties were used to diagnose diabetes because the ants are attracted by a sugar in urine (Lockhart, 2007). In Australia stinging inzula ants were used to treat colds and impotence in men, whereas in Morocco it was recommended to feed on ants for lethargy (Lockhart, 2007). Sore eyes and weak vision were treated with ant eggs mixed with an equal amount of white flour to make dough. The dough was lightly baked, mixed with red wine and put over closed eyes. Arabs used ants externally for leprosy and as an aphrodisiac. The main use of ants in Central Asia was in curing arthritis. In Russia bottles were filled half with ants and half with vodka and were kept in a warm place for several days. A teaspoonful of prepared remedy was taken morning and night to treat fever and other illnesses. For the treatment of paralysis live ants were tied in bags and were kept on the paralyzed part for 2-3 days (Lockhart, 2007).

Bees produce several valuable products important from nutritional and medicinal aspects. Honey, in addition to its high nutritional and culinary values, has antibacterial properties due to hydrogen peroxide that is produced continuously as a result of glucose-oxidizing enzyme that metabolizes glucose to gluconic acid and hydrogen peroxide. Propolis also exhibits high antibacterial activity.

Bee venom, a colorless liquid, also denoted as apitoxin, is produced by other insects as well. A honeybee can inject up to 0.1 mg of the venom via its stinger. It is estimated that about 1% of the population is allergic to bee sting. Bee venom causes local inflammation and acts as anticoagulant but can be deactivated with ethanol. The venom represents a complex mixture of proteins, including phospholipase which damages cell membranes and hyaluronidase (1-3%) which causes dilatation of capillaries. Histamine, which makes 0.5-2% of the venom, serves to increase permeability of capillaries to other active compounds in the venom. Besides histamine other biogenic amines are synthesized by bees including dopamine and noradrenalin which make about 1-2%. Protease-inhibitors which act as anti-inflammatory agents make about 2% of the venom. Adolapin from the venom (2-5%) has analgesic effects due to blocking of cyclooxygenase which is responsible for the formation of inflammatory mediators.

Bee stings were used since antiquity to treat various illnesses. The most potent anti-inflammatory agent in bee venom is melittin which is about hundred times more potent than hydrocortisol. In addition, melittin also induces the production of endogenous cortisol. The compound is composed of 62 amino acids and has several marked affects in addition to its anti-inflammatory character. By damaging mitochondrial membranes melittin provokes cell lysis. Apamin is another dominant protein in apitoxin that enhances nerve transmission in central nervous system by selective blocking of calcium-activated potassium channels, thus acting as a neurotoxin.

Therapeutic properties of bee venoms were recognized early in the history and already ancient Greek and Roman doctors, Hippocrates, Celsus, Galen and Pliny, described bee therapy for treating toothache, sore gums and dysentery. Both live and boiled bees were used in medical and veterinary practices as diuretic, to treat cough and for other therapeutic purposes. It is believed that the Holy Roman emperor Charlemagne was cured from gout by bee stings. Amazonian tribes used bees to determine if a person was dead, or in coma, because bees wouldn't sting a corpse and there wouldn't be any inflammation.

There was a reported case in the London hospital that revealed the possibility of using bees for treating alcoholism (Lockhart, 2007). The effects were discovered by accident after the patients have lost a desire for alcohol following bee stings. Efficiency of bee venom in treating skin conditions was also discovered accidentally when a beekeeper suffering from severe eczema was attacked by the bees. Skin area covered with eczema was significantly reduced afterwards (Lockhart, 2007). Antirheumatic effects of bee venom were frequently reported. Bee sting remarkably reduced both pain and swelling in patients suffering from arthritis and other systemic inflammations (Burt, 1937) After several doctors in Russia have found that bee stings could treat malaria, researches confirmed that finding on transgenic mosquitoes indicating that phospholipases from a venom are responsible for such effect (Moreira et al., 2002). The use of bee venom is also interesting in cosmetics and bee venom-based cosmetic products are nowadays available for treating scar tissues and to plump the lips or to initiate collagen production in the skin.

A first pharmaceutical product based on bee venom was produced in Egypt under the name Forapin in the mid 1930s. Forapin was prescribed for treating neuritis, sciatica and neuralgia. Later on an isolated fraction of bee venom with the estimated molecular weight of 1940 g/mol became available under the name Cardiopep, which stands for cardioactive peptide. The drug acts like a potent, nontoxic beta-adrenergic-like stimulant possessing definite anti-arrhythmic properties. The compound stabilizes heart rate and provides an increase in the strength of heart contractions. The product is recommended for irregular heart beat. Today also a tablet form of bee venom is available for treating rheumatism. In fact, different bee venom-based pharmaceutical preparations are available, however one should be aware that none of these products, not even injectable bee venom, can be as efficient as natural bee stings.

There are more than five hundreds species of **beetles-bombardiers** which produce irritant venom containing apitoxin, hydroquinone, hydrogen peroxide and other active compounds. Historically the insect gained popularity because Napoleon's soldiers crossing Pyrenees were attacked by it and were injured. The venom of beetles-bombardiers is a colorless, clear, bitter liquid with a pleasant smell. The insect stores hydroquinone and hydrogen peroxide in separate reservoirs of the body which come into a mixing chamber containing water and a mixture of catalytic enzymes. When the insect is felt threatened the compounds undergo exothermic chemical reaction, raising the temperature to near 100°C and expelling the produced venom from the anus (Blum, 1978). The symptoms of poisoning with beetles-bombardiers venom are highly dependent on skin location that was exposed to the venom. The venom of beetles-bombardiers was used in the treatment of rheumatism.

The **Spanish fly** lives throughout southern Europe, Central Asia and Siberia. In the past the insect was used as an ingredient in love potions and for sexual arousal, mostly for women. The insect produces venom that acts like an irritant to the urinary tract and sexual organs. This feeling was mistaken for a sexual desire where, in fact, it was an inflammation of sexual organs in question.

Bioactive and toxic compound of the Spanish fly venom is cantharidin (Figure VII.4), a terpenoid that is also produced by other insect species. The body of the beetle contains up to 5% of a fatty liquid cantharidin. In skin contact cantharidin causes reddening and rash, forming blisters.

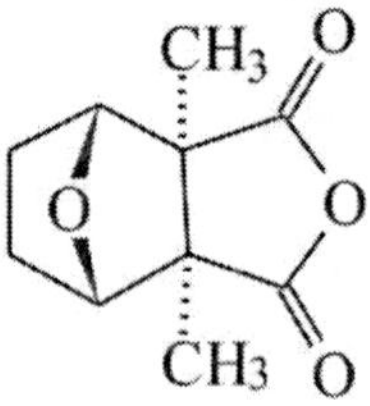

Figure VII.4. Cantharidin.

In the Renaissance period cantharidin was a component of *Aqua toffana*, a famous poison sold by professional poisoners to commit a murder. The mixture was composed of arsenic and cantharidin, and just 4 to 6 drops of a poison could lead to a slow death. After ingestion, distribution throughout the body and biotransformation, cantharidin is excreted in urine. During urination excreted metabolites cause irritation of the urogenital tract which leads to itching and swelling of the genitals. As a consequence kidneys may be permanently damaged. In veterinary practice cantharidin is sometimes given to farm animals to initiate the feelings of mating.

As a vesicant cantharidin has important place in the treatment of benign epithelial growths and for wart removal. In wart removal it is important not to leave the scar, and this gives prevalence to using cantharidin in comparison to other treatments.

In wart removal cantharidin is used when other treatments such as salicylic acid or cryotherapy are unsuccessful. Cantharidin is also effective in treating viral warts. Even not yet approved by FDA cantharidin is quite effective for wart treatment with efficiency of 33% after a single treatment. The procedure consists of covering the wart with cantharidin and bandaging it for 4-6h. After this period the compound is washed with a soap and water. When formed blister dries the wart comes off with the skin. Formed blister lifts the skin with the wart affecting only the dermal layer, and leaving a basal layer intacked, therefore not leaving scars. Cantharidin therapy should never be applied on moles, birthmarks, and undiagnosed skin lesions, nor on mucose membranes. In genital and anal area cantharidin therapy must be applied with great precaution.

4. VENOMS OF MARINE ORGANISMS

The number of venomous marine organisms is very vast and in last several decades more than 20,000 bioactive compounds have been isolated from sea organisms, such as corals, jellyfish, snails and others. According to extensive overview of different chemicals originating from different marine organisms it is clear that the complexity of the venom structure is independent on the developmental level of the organism. Marine microorganisms are another particularly rich source of new bioactive compounds.

Marine sponges are important sources of medicinally important bioactive compounds. Approximately 30% of all potential marine-derived medications and about 75% of recently patented marine-derived anticancer compounds originate from marine sponges. Discovery of spongothymidine in Caribbean sponge (*Cryptotethya crypta)* led to the development of a whole class of drugs for the treatment of cancer and viral diseases, such as Zidovudine for HIV positive patients and Acyclovir for the treatment of eczema and some herpes viruses.

Cone snail venoms are known under the term conotoxins. There are over 500 species of cone snails, each producing about hundred different conotoxins. In general, conotoxins are small peptide molecules composed of 12-30 amino acids and highly constrained due to dense disulphide bonds. Conotoxins are among the most potent and diverse neurotoxins known. There are three main classes of paralytic conotoxins α, μ and ω, acting by different mechanisms, by inhibiting nicotinic acetylcholine receptors, binding to postsynaptic sodium channels or by blocking of calcium entry (Han, 2008).

In envenomation with cone snail venoms the composition of the venom, as well as biological activity and symptoms of envenomation, are different with each injection. Cone snails deliver their venom through a stinger causing a swelling and intense pain in sting area. After swelling diminishes scars and blisters usually develop. Envenomation with conotoxins is accompanied with weakness, loss of coordination, and disruption of vision, speech and hearing. For envenomation with conotoxins there are no antivenoms developed, but as a part of the treatment tetanus prophylaxis may be useful.

Magician cone (*Conus magus*) produces venoms that show much promise for providing a non-addictive potent analgesics, whose potency is estimated to be thousand times more powerful than morphine (Han, 2008). The venom of Queen Victoria cone (*Conus victoriae*) accelerates the recovery from nerve injury and is effective in treating post surgical and neuropathic pain. Ziconotide (Prialt), approved by FDA in 2004, is the first analgesic derived from cone snail toxin.

The number of identified conotoxins counts in matter of hundreds, however only six conotoxins are currently undergoing clinical trials, and four are in a pre-clinical stage. Trials are oriented towards investigation of the venom efficiency in the treatment of Alzheimer's, Parkinson's diseases and epilepsy.

5. ANTIVENOMS

In envenomation treatment the most effective therapy implies administration of *antivenoms*, however the number of available antivenoms is limited. Antivenom is a biological product used in the treatment of venomous bites or stings that is mostly administrated intravenously, with the exception of envenomation by a stonefish or a redbeck spider when the antivenom is given intramuscularly. The principle of antivenom is, on oppose to vaccines where the immunity is induced directly in the patient, to induce immunological response in the antibody-producing host animal. Produced antibodies are further separated from animal plasma to produce antivenom. Produced antivenoms can be monovalent that are effective against a given species venom, or polyvalent, effective against a range of species venoms. In general, produced antivenoms are more efficient for neurotoxins, because they are produced in lesser quantities and are distributed to target tissues with a delay.

Administration of antivenoms may provoke immediate hypersensitivity reaction (anaphylaxis) or delayed hypersensitivity reaction, known as serum sickness, due to presence of host-animal serum proteins. Ideal antivenom would be possible to produce synthetically to avoid allergic reactions. In addition, ideal antivenom would be possible to administrate orally and would be equally efficient against a wide range of venoms. Ideal venom, however, doesn't exist and those are still being produced by immunizing host animals.

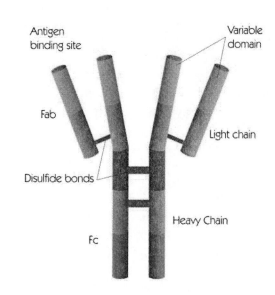

Figure VII.5. The structure of the antibody.

The animals, horses for large scale production, or sheep, goats and rabbits, are immunized with increasing doses of venom for prolonged period lasting up to a year. Antibody response in the animal is monitored in regular time intervals. After sufficient quantity of the antibodies has been produced the blood is collected and immunoglobulin's of a G class (IgG) are separated, purified and subjected to digestion into Fab fragments (Figure VII.5). Immunoglobulin's G (IgG) have a dominant role in antigen counteraction, however until sufficient quantity is produced IgM are taking over a role as first responders.

In human body there are five classes of antibodies, each having a distinct function. Antibodies of an A class (IgA) are abundantly produced in mucous tissues of gastrointestinal, respiratory and urogenital tract, where they prevent colonization by pathogens. Immunoglobulin's of a D class (IgD) are bound to the membranes of B cells playing a role of antigen receptors. In parasitic infections major responders are IgE, which in normal circumstances make only a small portion (~0.05%) of the circulating antibodies (Švarc-Gajić, 2009). This class of antibodies is also responsible for histamine release from mastocytes in allergic reactions.

Antibodies are Y shaped globulin molecules composed of two light and two heavy chains with both having constant and variable domains. Variable domains change with the activation of B cells by different antigens. Light and heavy chains are bound via disulphide bonds. Antibody interacts with the antigen via its Fab (Fragment antigen binding) fragments, whereas it's Fc (Fragment crystallizable) end serves for its adherence to cell membranes. Formed antigen/antibody complex can precipitate and be subjected to phagocytosis or may stimulate other paths of immunological response such as complement system.

Trends in antivenoms production imply *in vitro* techniques using human cells. Such approach would solve many problems related to antivenom therapy, however it is still being at the research level. Alternative solution would be to base the antivenom on avian yolk immunoglobulin's (IgY), which are principal antibodies in birds, reptiles, and lungfish. Immunoglobulin's of Y class are also found in high concentrations in chicken egg yolk and are functionally similar to mammalian IgG. Antivenoms based on avian yolk immunoglobulin's (IgY) would be less expensive, safer and more robust. Other possibility of improving the safety of antivenoms is to use sheep and rabbit immunoglobulin's which showed to be less allergenic. These differences in immunoreactivity are still not clear and remain to be investigated. Using smaller animals like rabbits require much more labor and expenses and this should be taken into account for large scale antivenom production.

REFERENCES

Blum, MS. Biochemical defenses of insects, 459-539. In: *Biochem ins*, Ed: Rockstein M. New York, Academic Press, 1978.

Burt JB. Bee venom therapy in chronic rheumatic disorder. *British J Phys Med* 171, 1937, 171-179.

Deshane J, Garner CC, Sontheimer H. Chlorotoxin inhibits glioma cell invasion via matrix metalloproteinase-2. *J Biol Chem* 278 (6), 2003, 4135–4144.

Fry BG, Wickramaratna JC, Hodgson WC, Winkel K, Wuster W. *J Toxicology-Toxin Rev.* 22(1), 2003, 23–34.

Han TS, Teichert RW, Olivera BM, Bulaj G. Conus Venoms - a Rich Source of Peptide-Based Therapeutics. *Currt Pharml Design.* 14, 2008, 2462-2479.

Lockhart GJ. *Ants, and other great medicines.* Unpublished book available on line from 2007.

Marsten Jl, Chan kok-ewe B. Ankeney Jl, Botti, R Bishop G, Bishop G. Antithrombotic Effect of Malayan Pit Viper Venom on Experimental Thrombosis of the Inferior Vena Cava Produced by a New Method. *Circ Res.* 19, 1966, 514-519.

McArdle JJ, Lentz TL, Witzemann V, Schwarz H, Weinstein SA, Schmidt JJ. Waglerin-1 selectively blocks the epsilon form of the muscle nicotinic acetylcholine receptor. *J Pharm Exp Ther* 289(1), 1999, 543-550.

Moreira LA, Ito J, Ghosh A, Devenport M, Zieler H, Abraham EG, Crisanti A, Nolan T, Catteruccia F, Jacobs-Lorena M. Bee Venom Phospholipase Inhibits Malaria Parasite Development in Transgenic Mosquitoes. *J Biol Chem* 277(43), 2002, 40829-40843.

Raufman JP, Jensen RT, Sutliff VE, Pisano JJ, Gardner JD. Actions of Gila monster venom on dispersed acini from guinea pig pancreas. *Am J Physiol.* 242(5), 1982, 470-474.

Švarc-Gajić, J. General Toxicology. Nova Science Publishers, New York, 2009.

Swenson S, Costa F, Minea R, Sherwin RP, Ernst W, Fujii G, Yang D, Markland FS . Intravenous liposomal delivery of the snake venom disintegrin contortrostatin limits breast cancer progression. *Mol Cancer Ther* 3(4), 2004, 499-511.

Veal DA.Antimicrobial properties of secretions from the metapleural glands of *Myrmecia gulosa* – the Australian Bullet ant. *J Appl Bact* 72, 1992, 188-192.

Zhou Q, Sherwin RP, Parrish C, Richters V, Groshen SG, Tsao-Wei D, Markland FS. Contortrostatin, a dimeric disintegrin from Agkistrodon contortrix contortrix, inhibits breast cancer progression. *Breast Cancer Res Treat.* 61(3), 2000, 249-260.

Chapter VIII

CHEMOMETRY OF NATURAL COMPOUNDS

Chemometry is a relatively new multidisciplinary science that in past several decades occupies the interest of scientists from different fields. First time this term was mentioned in 1971 as a Swedish word, but soon has got accepted by broad scientific community (Sharaf et al., 1986). The International Chemometrics Society (ICS) was established soon upon the term was coined defining it more specifically as "the science of relating measurements made on a chemical system or process to the state of the system via application of mathematical or statistical methods". More specifically elaborated, it can be said that chemometry extracts the information's from multivariate chemical systems using tools statistical and mathematical tool. Chemometry relates the results of measurements performed on chemical systems or processes with their properties by using computational modeling.

In analytical chemistry it is important to apply multivariate approach because experimental data, which in analytical chemistry may consider UV/VIS, IR, NMR spectra, chromatogram or other, are highly multivariate by their nature and their data sets may include up to 10 000 variables. Chemometric multivariate calibration techniques, such as principal component analysis (PCA) or partial last square regression (PLS), allow the definition of models that relate multivariate response (spectra, chromatogram) to concentration or any other property of interest.

Today chemometry is heavily used in analytical chemistry and metabolomics, but also this scientific discipline very successfully addresses problems in chemistry, biochemistry, medicine, biology and chemical engineering, by interlacing with disciplines such as multivariate statistics, applied mathematics, and computer science.

Independently on the area that it is applied on, the procedure of chemometric analysis relies on two important steps, data collection and information derivation by implying advanced statistical analysis or pattern recognition and exploiting computer technology. Because this scientific discipline implies advanced computer technologies, before their development to sufficient level that enabled mathematical and statistical manipulation with large sets of data, chemometry was virtually impossible to exist.

Chemometry can be observed from many facets and can also be described as a form of descriptive or predictive chemistry. In *descriptive* approach properties of chemical systems are modeled with the intent of defining relationships within the systems. In *predictive* applications, properties of chemical systems are modeled with the final aim of predicting properties or behavior of other system elements or predicting properties other of those used in modeling.

Many chemometric models, both descriptive and predictive, rely on molecular descriptors. *Molecular descriptors* are numerical data describing specific molecular property and are defined by mathematical calculations or experimentally. Modern softwares and mathematical programs allow calculation of more than two thousands molecular descriptors, whereas first commercial softwares were able to calculate only about two hundred. These softwares integrate the knowledge on algebra, informatics, physical chemistry and statistics. Application of numerical data for describing specific molecular property allows more straightforward definition of the quantitative relationship between the molecular structure, physico-chemical properties and biological activity. Furthermore, this makes the prediction and estimation of specific molecular property more accurate. For a single molecule there is unlimited number of possible molecular descriptors. By using numerical designators different molecular properties, such as lipophilicity, ability to form hydrogen bonds, some electronical (charge, polarizability, dipole moment, energy state), sterical or topological characteristics, can be expressed objectively.

Molecular descriptors vary according to complexity of information's they provide. One-dimensional (1D) descriptors are the simplest and may include, e.g. molecular bruto formula. Two-dimensional (2D) molecular descriptors are calculated on the basis of two-dimensional molecular structure, while three-dimensional (3D) require 3D molecular presentation. The examples of 2D and 3D molecular descriptors include topological indexes or complex molecular properties such as refraction, respectively. Pharmacokinetic data are modeled on the basis of 3D descriptors because they consider complex spatial interactions with receptors. Table 1 lists some of the triazine molecular descriptors.

Table 1. Some of the triazine molecular descriptors.

	Molecule	Descriptor
1D	C17H28ClN5	Molecular mass Atomic descriptors
2D		Fragment contribution Topological indexes Connectivity Flexibility
3D		Molecular surface Molecular volume Energy of interaction Valence characteristics Wave characteristics

Frequently applied chemometric models heavily relying on molecular descriptors include Quantitative Structure Property Relationship (QSPR), Quantitative Structure Activity Relationship (QSAR) and Quantitative Structure Retention Relationship (QSRR) (Massart et al., 1988). QSPR models are mathematical models linking chemical structure to the specific property, whereas QSAR models define the relationship between the structure and biological activity. These models are very useful because it is much easier to synthesize compound of preset chemical structure than of preset property, and especially with the development in organic chemistry and improvement in analytical tools that enabled reliable identification, this task became straightforward. Mathematical models for predicting molecular properties on the basis of chromatographic behavior, both in laminar and column chromatographic techniques, are known as QSRR.

1. QSPR MODELS

Physical properties, such as color, density, electrical conductivity, melting point, etc., are related to molecular structure, but chemical reactivity and biological activity are also structure-dependent. To some instance this chemometric model can be observed as a combinatorial model where chemometric approaches relaying on molecular descriptors are interlaced. To obtain good correlations it is of utmost importance to choose adequate molecular descriptors.

Chemometric models relating molecular structure with the property highly support the trends in analytical chemistry to develop simple and rapid techniques that allow direct analysis. Some analytical techniques rely on the existence of such dependence, such as Near Infrared Transmission (NIT) spectroscopy, or Near Infrared Reflection (NIR) spectroscopy. In these techniques reflection or transmission of the near infrared light of the native sample is measured at great number of selected wavelengths. The intensity of molecular transmission or reflection in near infrared range is dependent on the chemical composition of the sample, i.e. on the molecules present in the sample. In order to correlate measured light intensity with structure-dependent parameter, usually to the content of specific molecules, like proteins, water or fats, these system require thorough calibration with input data of large sets of reference samples in which the desired information (protein content e.g.) is produced by some reference technique. Calibration is made for each sample type individually defining the representative or reference behavior of the systems in respect to desired information. In these analytical techniques calibration step is the most time consuming and tedious. After proper calibration these models, i.e. analytical techniques, allow analyst to obtain required information's in matter of minutes by direct sample analysis, avoiding its preparation. Direct analysis enables numerous benefits, such as reduction in time, energy and chemicals consumption, and avoidance of sample preparation step, reducing the risks of sample contamination and analyte loss. These elegant analytical techniques, however, could not have existed before computational techniques were sufficiently developed to allow multivariate modeling.

2. QSRR MODELS

To be reliable models linking specific chemical structure, molecular bioactivity or specific property, to chromatographic behavior, require input of adequate data and correct statistical analysis. The models are applicable for great number of input data obtained under constant conditions, i.e. are useful in the analysis of complex mixtures composed of great number of solutes. To be reliable these models analyzing simultaneously numerous molecules, require sufficient number of molecular descriptors. QSRR correlations can be used for predictive purposes only if proved to be statistically significant, i.e. if developed models show good correlations with assumed dependences. Under such terms QSRR correlations can be used for different purposes (Figure VIII.1), such as elucidation of chromatographic processes that can be used in identification of unknown solutes, prediction of chromatographic behavior, elucidation of retention mechanisms on a molecular level, or for comparison of different stationary phases. The models may be implied to predict biological activity within series of related compounds and to estimate complex molecular characteristics such as lipophilicity, dissociation constant, etc. According to calculated correlations and statistical significance of the developed models for different molecular designators, descriptors that best describe relevant molecular information's can be selected. Poorly correlated models can lead to inaccurate conclusions. Being simple to conduct, as well as due to simple collection of experimental data, the models are frequently used in analytical, clinical and physical chemistry.

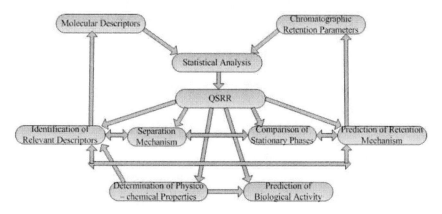

Figure VIII.1. Application of QSRR models.

3. LIPOPHILICITY IN ADME (ABSORPTION, DISTRIBUTION, METABOLISM, EXCRETION) AND QSRR MODELS

In 1941 Martin with the coworkers demonstrated that retention parameterscan be successfully correlated to lipophilicity of the compounds, i.e. to logP. Distribution between lipophylic and hydrophilic phases occurs not only in chromatography but also in biological systems and processes accompanying xenobiotic from the entrance into the body to its elimination. Lipophilicity of molecules is important for the passage across cell membranes, a process that is in the core of all major toxicokinetic/pharmacokinetic steps, i.e. absorption, distribution, metabolism and excretion (ADME) (Figure VIII.2). Consequently, it can be assumed that chromatographic behavior, i.e. lipophilicity (logP), may correlate well with the ability to pass biological membranes and barriers (van de Waterbeemd and Gifford, 2003).

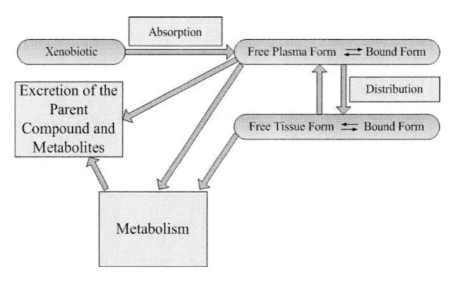

Figure VIII.2. Toxicokinetic/pharmacokinetic processes occurring in the body.

Lipophilicity expressed in terms of logP values is one of the most important molecular parameters in QSRR. Today around twenty softwares for calculating different variations of logP values are available. This parameter is valuable and is used in medical chemistry and molecular pharmacology but is, however, only the rough estimate of the molecular chemical nature.

LogP value represents the logarithm of concentrations ratio in octanol (C_o), as highly hydrophobic medium, and water (C_w):

$$\log P = \log \frac{C_O}{C_W}$$

The greater the partition coefficient is (P), the molecule is considered to be more lipophylic. Range of partition coefficients for molecules of significantly different polarities is too wide, so logarithmic values are taken as measures of the molecular character. In biological environment more applicable would be to observe distribution ratio (D) which takes into account total concentration of the compound, including all its forms. This is important if the compound undergoes some secondary reactions in one of the phases, such as dissociation or complex formation. For biological processes mostly distribution ratio values at pH 7.4 and 6.5 are important, which simulate, respectively, blood and gut conditions.

Even though lipophilicity and hydrophobicity are often used interchangeably, according to IUPAC they have different meaning. Thus "lipophilicity" is the "affinity of molecules or molecular parts toward lipophilic surrounding expressed through the partition coefficient in two-phase liquid/liquid system, whereas "hydrophobicity" is defined as "joining of non-polar functionalities or molecules in aqueous surrounding due to tendency of the water molecules to remove non-polar molecules".

In some cases the correlation of retention parameters with logP values can be moderate because partitioning and chromatographic systems differ. Immobilized liquid phases in chromatographic systems have one degree of freedom less, acting different in comparison to bulk liquids. In chromatographic techniques proportionally smaller volumes of liquid phases are used. Possible interactions make chromatographic processes distinct in comparison to sole distribution between two immiscible phases:

- Solute/stationary phase interactions
- Solute/mobile phase interactions
- Stationary phase/mobile phase interactions
- Interactions between molecular flexible fragments of the stationary phase

Octanol is convenient for the modeling of the distribution across cell membranes because the solvent can be both the donor and the acceptor of hydrogen atoms, same as the phospholipids in membranes. Other non-polar solvents can be used to model molecular lipophilicity. Distribution, thus, is observed in systems chloroform/water, alkane/water or propylene-glycol-dipelargonate/water. In classical approach to calculate logP values the compound is shaken in the system composed of two immiscible solvents. After equilibration and phase separation, concentrations are measured in both phases and logP is subsequently calculated. Problems associated with traditional method of calculating partition coefficient are related to necessity to control temperature accurately and to estimation of the minimal solvent volume that will be used in the assay. Furthermore, octanol has unpleasant smell and forms emulsions. To avoid emulsion formation the system can be gently stirred during equilibration. The procedure is long lasting and cannot be used for solutes that dissociate or have logP>6.

Indirect methods for calculating logP values include:

- Reverse phase chromatography
- Micellar electrokinetic chromatography
- Potentiometric method - pH
- Filter probe measurement

Reverse phase chromatography provides advantages of being rapid and cheap, and not requiring quantitation. The method isn't, however, adequate for chlorinated hydrocarbons, nor for compounds with low logP. If silica-based plates/columns are used acidity range is limited to 2-7.5 due to instability of the silica backbone and hydrolysis of bonds with alkyl chains. Micellar electrokinetic chromatography uses surfactants above critical micellar concentrations. The method is used for neutral molecules that in the form of micelles can be separated in the electrical field. The method is not applicable for molecules that dissociate. For ionized molecules potentiometric method is recommended. Two titrations in the method are performed. The first one is carried out with 0.5 M KOH until high pH is reached. After octanol addition second titration is completed with 0.5 M HCl until starting pH. For lipophilic substances second titration curve will differ from the first one. For molecules with high logP values the difference between two equivalence points is great. Filter probe measurement is similar to potentiometric method but the detection is spectrometric. The method is rapid, reliable, but is not recommended for substances with logP<0.2, and may give inaccurate results for charged, ionized or tautomeric molecules, zwitter ions and molecules that form strong hydrogen bonds.

As a measure of chromatographic hydrophobicity parameters, QSRR models rely on $logk_w$, in column techniques, or on R_{m0} in laminar chromatographic techniques, obtained by extrapolation to zero volume fraction of organic solvent in the mobile phase (φ):

$$\log k = \log k_w + S\phi$$
$$R_m = R_{m_0} + S\phi$$

S is the slope of the dependences, a constant specific to the system of particular solute, stationary and mobile phase. $log\ k$ and R_m values are calculated on the basis of retention parameters in chromatography:

$$\log k = \log(\frac{1}{t_r} - 1)$$
$$R_m = \log(\frac{1}{R_f} - 1)$$

By extrapolating to zero molar fraction of the organic solvent the influence of the solvent type is eliminated. These parameters ($log\ K_w$, R_{m0}) are virtual because such situation would not allow good separation of the compounds.

Besides linear models correlating R_m or $log\ K_w$ with the molar fraction of organic solvent, square model can also be used:

$$R_m = A\phi^2 + B\phi + R_{m_0}$$
$$\log K_w = A'\phi^2 + B'\phi + \log K_w$$

A, A', B and B' are constants characteristic for the systems. In general, better correlations are obtained with the linear model, however for methanol the difference for two models is insignificant, therefore for lipophilicity determination methanol should be the solvent of choice.

4. *IN SILICO* MODELING

Traditional drug development included compound synthesis and pre-clinical *in vitro* and *in vivo* studies to determine whether such compound can be considered a candidate for clinical trial. It is not a rare case that candidates selected in pre-clinical assays in later stages of drug testing demonstrate lack of efficiency, poor pharmacokinetics, animal toxicity or expressed adverse effects in humans. Compounds with unsatisfactory pharmacological profile must be rejected even though years of interdisciplinary endeavor and billions of dollars have been invested. To avoid such unfortunate scenario frequently seen in traditional approach of drug development novel methodologies are being proposed. Modern process of drug development is based on combinatorial chemistry, genomics, HTP (High Throughput Screening), chemometrics and *in silico* processing. *In silico* modeling refers to modeling performed on a computer or via computer simulation. By this computational approach the failure in drug development is reduced to a minimum. Developed models, defined by using large series of related compounds, serve to forecast the behavior in biological systems and to predict biological activity of the compounds related to ones used in the modeling. In this way derivatives with advanced pharmacological profile can be anticipated, further synthesized and subjected to *in vitro*, *in vivo* tests, and examined clinically. In HTP (High Throughput Screening) large sets of available compounds are roughly screened on test plates for their bioactivity using robotic systems, further selecting potential candidates.

The term *in silico* was coined in 1989 with the analogy to commonly used scientific Latin phrases *in vivo, in vitro, in situ* etc. In this modern approach the programs perform calculations to produce desired information's based on the molecular structure. Where one group of these computational methods focuses on toxicodynamic and biological activity, trying to forecast interactions with target receptors, others tend to predict the fate of the substance in the human body, i.e. absorption, distribution, metabolism and excretion (ADME). Toxicodynamic/pharmacodynamic aspects that are normally anticipated by *in silico* modeling include the ability to bind to plasma proteins (PPB - Plasma Protein Binding), the ability to cross blood/brain barrier (BBB - Blood Brain Barrier) and bioavailability in the digestive tracts (HIA - Human Intestinal Absorption). Plasma protein binding represents the ratio of bound concentration and total plasma concentration, expressed in %. Good human intestinal absorption is important for drugs intended for oral administration and is calculated as:

HIA = ((oral dose – excreted concentration)/oral dose) x100

Pharmacodynamic properties that are most often computationally predicted include *in silico* estimation of the compounds ability to act as:

- Nuclear receptor ligand
- Ion channel modulator
- GPCR (G-Protein Coupled Receptor) ligand
- Kinase inhibitor
- Enzyme inhibitor
- Protease inhibitor

Nuclear receptors are important because they control metabolic processes, whereas ion channels maintain membrane potential. G–proteins are located at the inner membrane surface (Figure VIII.3) connecting the receptors with effector proteins that further signal intracellular processes. Protein-kinases encompass more than 500 molecular proteins in the cell and are very important in regulating signal transmission in the cell. These proteins regulate majority of cellular pathways by phosphorilating other proteins. Phosphorylation usually results in changing enzyme activity, cellular location, or association with other proteins. Because each phosphate group carries two negative charges, the addition of one phosphate group causes a change in the shape of a protein. Altered protein shape is often correlated with altered activity of the protein. Thus, the ability to change conformation of the protein between two different shapes allows the control of protein's activity. Phosphorylation by kinases is a reversible process, and proteins are dephosphorylated by phosphatases. Harmonized activity of protein kinases and phosphatases initiate and stop major cellular events according to cellular requirements. Among many cellular events kinases are responsible for the control of cell growth and cell division. Cell growth and cell cycle pathways are activated in cancer cells, so the cells continue to divide even in the absence of external signals like those from growth factors. Growth factors are excreted by other cells subsequently binding to receptors on the cell surface, stimulating cell division. In cancerous cells division is not regulated adequately and one of the reasons could be a mutation in a kinase or phosphatase gene, leading to proliferation of the cancerous cells (Blume-Jensen and Hunter, 2004).

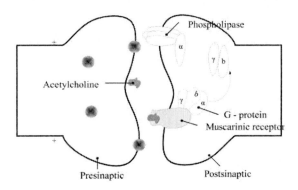

Figure VIII.3. G-protein coupled receptors in synapses.

To estimate whether potentially attractive pharmaceutical compound is adequate for oral administration, Lipinski`s rule of five is used. The molecule has a potential to be used as oral pharmaceutical if (Lipinski et al., 2001):

- M<500 Da
- log Kow<5
- The number of hydrogen bond donors: <5
- The number of hydrogen bond acceptors: <10 (nitrogen or oxygen atoms)

All numbers are multiples of five, which is the root of the rule's name. Potential candidates for oral pharmaceuticals are further subjected to generation of ADME data by *in vitro* assays, *in silico* or predictive models.

Two popular on-line softwares that allow calculation of molecular properties and prediction of their bioactivity are Molinspiration and ChemSilico. The first one can be attained by entering the web address http://www.molinspiration.com. For software to be able to calculate some specific molecular descriptors and biological predictors, a three-dimensional molecular structure is required. Molecular structure can be uploaded or can be generated directly on-line in a provided window. In Molinspiration program generated three-dimensional molecular structure can be rotated and presented in selected way. Polar surface area, numbers of rotational bonds, molecular volume, milogP, are just some of the common molecular descriptors calculated by Molinspiration. The program also allows virtual screening of the biological compatibility of newly synthesized compounds in respect to kinase inhibition, binding to nuclear receptors, ion channel modulation, etc.

In silico calculated molecular descriptors and predictors for natural bioactive compounds allow objective comparison of their properties and biological activity (Tables VIII.2 and VIII.4). According to calculated descriptors it can be concluded that natural carotenoids have similar polarities and no polar surface area, except for zeaxanthin, which belongs to xanthophyll class. As a demonstration, in Tables VIII.2 and VIII.4 are given calculated molecular descriptors and predictors for natural carotenoids.

The programmes that allow *in silico* calculation of biological predictors can be used for drug modeling and prediction of the biological activity of derivatives. Discovered natural bioactive compounds often in addition to desired biological effect exhibit some adverse effects or poor pharmacokinetic. To predict in which direction organic synthesis should precede, prior chemical transformation and biological tests, potential candidates can be subjected to calculation of their biological activity predictors. If β-carotene, e.g., is a parent compound on which other synthetic or semisynthetic biologically active compounds will be based on, depending on the desired property, different substitutions can be tested (Table VIII.3).

According to calculated molecular descriptors derivative 3 (Table VIII.4) has the highest molecular polar surface area (TPSA), but already introduction of just one hydroxyl group (derivative 1) significantly changed TPSA. Even though all β-carotene derivatives are unpolar, the highest log P, i.e. the lowest polarity, was calculated in derivative 2.

According to calculated predictors among natural carotenoids there are no significant differences in respect to ion channel modulation or enzyme inhibition (Table VIII.4). Zeaxanthin is the strongest kinase inhibitor while beta-carotene has the strongest potential for binding to nuclear receptors. Delta – carotene has the highest potential for activating G-protein coupled receptors.

Among synthetic β-carotene derivatives the highest potential for binding to G-protein coupled receptors has derivative 3 in which two hydroxyl groups and alkyl functionalities have been introduced (Table VIII.5). The same derivative, however, has the lowest affinity for affecting ion channels, but highest kinase inhibiting ability. Overall interesting modification of the biological activity has been achieved in derivative 3. Parent compound, β-carotene, has a potential to act as a nuclear receptor ligand, however modified derivative 3, according to *in silico* predictors, shows a potential for avoiding such effect.

Table VIII.2. Molecular properties of carotenoids.

	Compound	Structure	Properties						
			miLogP	TPSA	natoms	MW	nrotb	volume
1	α-carotene		9.791	0.0	40.0	536.888	10	591.99
2	β-carotene		9.793	0.0	39.0	522.861	10	575.403
3	γ-carotene		9.912	0.0	40.0	536.888	13	596.917
4	δ-carotene		9.864	0.0	40.0	536.888	13	596.94

	Compound	Structure	Properties					
			miLogP	TPSA	natoms	MW	nrotb	volume
5	Lycopene		9.977	0.0	40.0	536.888	16	601.871
6	Zeaxantin		9.390	40.456	42.0	568.886	10	608.052

Table VIII.3. Molecular properties of β-carotene derivatives.

	Compound	Structure	Properties					
			miLogP	TPSA	natoms	MW	nrotb	volume
1	β-carotene		9.793	0.0	39.0	522.861	10	575.403

Table VIII.3. (Continued)

	Compound	Structure	Properties						
			miLogP	TPSA	natoms	MW	nrotb	volume
2	Derivative 1		9.734	20.228	41.0	552.887	10	600.008
3	Derivative 2		10.126	0.0	45.0	607.023	14	675.758
4	Derivative 3		9.55	43.694	48.0	654.036	12	703.635

Table VIII.4. *In silico* biological predictors for natural carotenoids.

	Compound	Structure	Bioactivity					
			GPCR ligand	Ion channel modulator	Kinase inhibitor	Nuclear receptor ligand	Protease inhibitor	Enzyme inhibitor
1	α-carotene		0.02	-0.14	0.14	0.49	0.12	0.27
2	β-carotene		0.04	-0.10	0.14	0.53	0.08	0.29
3	γ-carotene		0.01	-0.14	0.17	0.47	0.07	0.26
4	δ-carotene		0.13	-0.10	0.08	0.42	0.11	0.27

Table VIII.4. (Continued)

	Compound	Structure	Bioactivity					
			GPCR ligand	Ion channel modulator	Kinase inhibitor	Nuclear receptor ligand	Protease inhibitor	Enzyme inhibitor
5	Lycopene		0.07	-0.12	0.06	0.29	0.06	0.17
6	Zeaxantin		0.08	-0.36	0.24	0.35	0.01	0.13

Table VIII.5. *In silico* biological predictors of β-carotene derivatives.

Compound	Structure	Bioactivity					
		GPCR ligand	Ion channel modulator	Kinase inhibitor	Nuclear receptor ligand	Protease inhibitor	Enzyme inhibitor
1 β-carotene		0.04	-0.10	0.14	0.53	0.08	0.29
2 Derivative 1		0.03	-0.28	0.18	0.38	0.12	0.27
3 Derivative 2		0.15	-0.64	0.50	0.16	0.18	0.03

Table VIII.5. (Continued)

Compound	Structure	Bioactivity					
		GPCR ligand	Ion channel modulator	Kinase inhibitor	Nuclear receptor ligand	Protease inhibitor	Enzyme inhibitor
4 Derivative 3		0.41	-1.04	0.85	-0.36	0.25	0.39

ChemSilico softwares, available on-line at http://chemsilico.com, allow calculation of total 519 topological and electronic-state descriptors. The user is required first to register on-line gaining the opportunity for free molecular characterization via different molecular descriptors for first twenty submitted structures. The results are sent to the e-mail of the registered user. On the basis of submitted molecular structure ChemSilico calculates molecular descriptors, such as logP, logD, logWS (water solubility), pKa and others. The program also provides several predictors, such as human intestinal absorption, penetration through blood/brain barrier, binding to plasma proteins and prediction of the outcome of the Ames mutagenicity test. In ChemSilico on-line software over 35,000 compounds were used to develop predictors using neural network and QSAR models.

REFERENCES

Blume-Jensen P and Hunter T. Oncogenic kinase signalling. *Nature*, 411(6835), 2001, 355-365.

Lipinski CA, Lombardo F, Dominy BW, Feeney PJ. Experimental and computational approaches to estimate solubility and permeability in drug discovery and development settings. *Adv Drug Del Rev* 46, 2001, 3–26.

Massart DL, Vandeginste BGM, Deming SM, Michotte Y, Kaufman L *Chemometrics: a textbook,* Elsevier 1988.

Sharaf MA, Illman DL, Kowalski BR. *Chemometrics*, Wiley, 1986.

van de Waterbeemd, H, Gifford E.ADMET in silico modeling: towards prediction paradise? *Nature Rev Drug Disc* 2, 2003, 192–204.

INDEX

#

β-glucuronidases, 23
1'- hydroxyestragole, 31
5-hydroxyindoleacetic acid, 52

A

Acetylcholine, 58, 63, 64, 66, 106, 110, 118, 121
Adrenaline, 22, 88, 89, 109
Agmantine, 88
Agonists, 24, 48, 95
Albumin, 14
Algae, 36, 40
Alkaloids, vi, ix, 37, 38, 57
Alveoli, 18
Antagonists, 24, 48
Antarease, 112
Antibody, 119, 120
Anticonvulsant, 46, 67
Antitumor effect, 82
Antivenoms, x, 107, 118, 119, 120
Antraquinones, 82, 83
Apitoxin, 114, 115, 116
Ayurvedic medicine, 27

B

Bacillus thuringiensis, 73
Batroxobin, 109
Bees, 114
Beetles-bombardiers, 116
Bioactive amines, 88
Bioactive substance, 14
Biogenic amines, 89
Blood/brain barrier, 14, 15, 62, 81, 89, 132, 142
Blood/brain barrier, 14
Botulinum toxin, 34, 110
Brucine, 63

C

Caffeic acid, 81
Caffeine, 61
Cannabinoids, 32
Cannabis sativa, 32
Cantharidin., 116
Capsaicin, 93, 94, 95
Capsaicinoids, 93
Cardiotonic glycosides, 30
Carotenoids, 53
Carpaine, 102, 103
Ceruroplasmine, 14
Chalcone, 75

Chavicine, 95
Chemometry, vii, x, 123, 124
Chinitases, 101
Chorionic Villus, 16
Chymopapain, 101
Ciguatoxin, 36
Clavinet type ergot alkaloids, 58, 59
Coagulation, 107
Codeine, 40
Competitive antagonists, 24
Conotoxins, 118
Contortrostatin, 110
Coumarin, 30
Curculin, 98
Cyanogenic glycosides, 30
Cycasin, 77
Cytochrome P450 oxidases, 21
Cytotrophoblasts, 16

D

Datura, 64, 65, 67
Deer antler velvet, 35
Diamine oxidase, 88
Dicoumarol, 31
Digitalis purpurea, 30
Djenkol, 90
Dopamine, 15, 58, 59, 61, 68, 88, 114
D-phenylalanine, 47, 55

E

Ecarin, 109
Elimination kinetics, 26
Endothelial cells, 15
Epibatidine, 112
Ergocryptine, 60, 68
Ergometrine, 60
Ergonovine, 59
Ergot alkaloids, 37, 57, 58
ergotamine, 38, 39, 59, 60, 68
Ergotamine, 38, 59, 60
Estragole, 31

F

Ferulic acid, 71, 82
Fibrin, 107, 109
Fibrinogen, 107, 109
Finger cherry, 97
First-pass effect, 17, 59
Flavanols, 70, 71, 72
Flavanones, 72
Flavin adenine dinucleotide (FAD), 22
Flavin-containing monooxygenase system, 21
Flavokavain B, 47
Flavonoids, 70, 71
Flavonols, 70, 71
Formic acid, 112, 113
Furocoumarins, 49, 55

G

Gangrene, 58, 61, 95
Ginkgo biloba L., 32
Ginkgolides, 32
Ginkgotoxin, 33, 43
Glial cells, 15
Gossypol, 73, 74, 84

H

Hematuria, 90
Hemitoxiferine, 62
Hepatotoxicity, 47, 55
Hippocrates, 28, 29, 115
Histamine-N- methyltransferase, 88
Homeopathy, v, 29
Hydrolytical enzymes, 23
Hydrophobicity, 129, 130, 131
Hydroxybenzoic Acid, 70
Hydroxytyrosol, 80, 81, 83
Hyperpigmentation, 49
Hypoglycine, 90, 91

I

Immunoglubulines, 120
In silico, x, 132, 133, 134, 135, 142
Iridomyrmecin, 112
Irreversible antagonists, 24
Isoflavonoids, 71, 72

K

Katemfe fruit, 98
Kava lactones, 46
Kava-kava, 46

L

Lathyrogens, 91, 92
Lignans, 70, 71, 72
Lipinski`s rule of five, 134
Lipophilicity, 128
Local effects, 14
LogP, 128, 129, 130, 142
Lovastatin, 34
L-phenylalanine, 48
LSD, 60, 61
Lutein, 53
Lycopene, 53, 54, 55, 137, 140

M

Marine sponges, 117
Meso-zeaxanthin, 53
Metabotropic receptors, 24
Methemoglobinemia, 18
Methysergide, 59
Miracle fruit, 98
Miraculin, 98
Molecular descriptors, 124
Mongolian medicine, 28
Monkeys' coconut, 92
Monoamine oxidase (MAO), 88
Monoamine oxygenases, 22
Morphine, 14, 39, 40, 41, 45, 64, 118

Morphine, 40
Moxibustion, 28
Multivariate calibration techniques, 123

N

Nabilone, 32
Narcotine, 40
Near Infrared Reflection (NIR)
    spectroscopy, 126
Neurolathyrogens, 91
Nociceptors, 95
Nux-Vomica alkaloids, 62

O

Oleuropein, 99, 100
Opium alkaloids, v, 39
Osteolathyrism, 92

P

Papain, 101
Papaverine, 40
Papaya, 100, 103
Paracelsus, 13
Parkinsonism, 48, 59, 60
Partial agonist, 24
Partition coefficient, 129, 130
p-Coumaric acid, 70
Peroxidases, 22
Persin, 97
Phase II reactions, 21, 23
Phenolic acids, 70
Phenolic compounds, x, 69, 83, 98, 99, 103
Phenylalanine, 47, 90
phenylethylamine, 47, 88
Phloretin, 76, 77
Phlorizin, 75, 76, 77, 84
Phototherapeutic agents, 49, 50
Phototoxic reactions, 49
Phytochemicals, 45
Phytoestrogens, 45, 48, 55, 72
Phytolaccigenin, 31

Phytolaccine, 31
Phytolaccotoxin, 31
Piperine, 95, 96, 104
Plant steroids, 30
Platelet-Aggregating Factor (PAF), 32
Pneumoconiosis, 19
Pokeweeds, 31
Pravastatin, 34
Prostaglandins, 70
Psoralens, 49, 50
Purine alkaloids, 61

Q

Quantitative Structure Activity
   Relationship(QSAR), 125
Quantitative Structure Property Relationship
   (QSPR), 125
Quantitative Structure Retention
   Relationship(QSRR), 125

R

Resiniferatoxin, 93
Resveratrol, 77, 79, 80, 84, 85, 86
Reversible antagonists, 24
Rhodomyrtoxins, 97

S

Safrole, 50, 51
SALT (skin associated lymphoid tissue), 19
Samuel Hahnemann, 29
Sassafras, 50, 51
Saxitoxin, 36
Scopolamine, 64
Scorpion, 112
Sedative, 67
Selenoaminoacids, 92
Serotonin, 22, 51, 52, 58, 59, 60, 61, 67, 68,
   88, 89
Siddha medicine, 28
Simvastin,, 34
Skin whitening, 31

Snake venoms, x, 106, 107, 109
Sodium-linked Glucose Transporters
   (SGLT), 76
Solanine, 65, 66, 67
Spanish fly, 116
St. Anthony's Fire, 58
Stilbene, 72
Stratum corneum, 20
Strychnine, 62, 63, 64
Strychnos Nux-vomica, 62
Syncytiotrophoblast., 16
Systematic effects, 14, 75, 87

T

Tacrolimus, 34, 35
Tebain, 40
Terpenophenolics, 32
Tetrodotoxin, 36
Thaumatins, 98
Theobromine, 62
Theophylline, 62
Tibetan medical system, 28
Tomatinase, 66
Tomatine, 65
Toxicodynamics, v, 23
Toxicokinetics, v, 25
Toxinology, 105
Traditional Chinese medicine, 28
Traditional medicine, v, 27
Transfferin,, 14
Transmembrane receptors, 24
Tropane alkaloids, 64
Trophoblastic cells, 16
TrpV1 receptors, 94
Two-compartment open model, 25
Tyramine, 88, 89

U

Unani medicine, 28

V

Venoms, vi, 105, 106, 121

W

Waglerin-1, 110

Z

zeaxanthin, 53, 135